FOCUS ON ARBOVIRUS INFECTIONS

FOCUS ON ARBOVIRUS INFECTIONS

VIROJ WIWANITKIT

Nova Biomedical Books
New York

Library of Congress Cataloging-in-Publication Data

Viroj Wiwanitkit.
Focus on arbovirus infections / Viroj Wiwanitkit.
p. ; cm.
Includes bibliographical references and index.
ISBN 978-1-60741-192-5 (hardcover)
1. Arbovirus infections. I. Title.
[DNLM: 1. Arbovirus Infections. WC 524 V819f 2009]
QR201.A72V57 2009
579.2'562--dc22 2009002392

Published by Nova Science Publishers, Inc. ✝ New York

Contents

Preface

Arthropod-borne disease is a common health problem all over the world. The term "arboviral diseases" refers to arthropod-borne arboviral infections. The purpose of this book is to summarize and present the topics specifically relating to the mosquito-borne disease that is unique to the tropical countries. Due to globalization in the present day, the change in the epidemiology of diseases from one site to the others all around the world can be expected. A summation of the common arboviral diseases can be and should be performed. This book can familiarize the reader with the problems. The book will cover specifically the clinical aspect, scientific laboratory aspect, public health aspect as well as the social sciences relating to important arboviral infectious diseases. The common arboviral diseases will be summarized, presented and discussed. The book will present summative data from the molecular to the population scales, as well as additional metanalysis of important topics. In addition, the diagnostic guideline and clinical practice guideline of the mentioned conditions will be presented. This work can be a useful reference for the practitioners who are not familiar with the unique problems of the developing world and might be faced with those problems due to the possible migration of diseases. The academic level of this book targets a wide range, from the medical student, resident, general practitioner, specialist in infectious and tropical medicine, and researcher in medical sciences. It can also be useful for medical personnel in allied health sciences.

Introduction to Arbovirus Infection

What Is Arbovirus Infection?

Infection is significant present-day concern. The disease carried by vector is an important group of contagious diseases. Arbovirus infection is group of arthropod-borne diseases in which the pathogenic microorganism is transmitted from an infected individual to another individual by an arthropod or other agent, sometimes with other animals serving as intermediary [1]. Basically, the transmission depends on attributes and the conditions of at least three different living organisms: a) the pathologic agent, the virus, the protozoan, the parasite or the bacteria; b) the vector, ordinarily arthropods such as ticks or mosquitoes; and c) the human or hosts [1-2]. Moreover, intermediary hosts, such as domesticated and wild animals, often serve as reservoirs for the pathogen until the susceptible human populations are exposed [1-2]. Arbovirus infection is a specific type of arthropod-borne disease in which the pathogen is a virus and there must be an arthropod vector to help transmit the disease. The principle for three compositions of epidemiology can be applied.

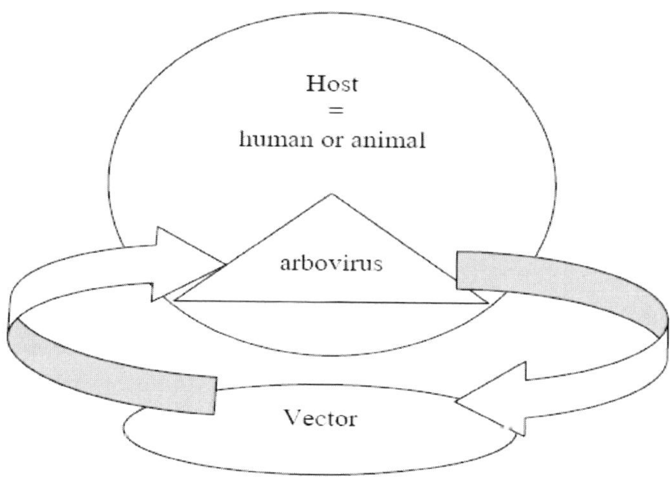

Wiwanitkit, 2005.

Figure 1. Mechanism of an arbovirus infection.

Of various arboviral illnesses, the mosquito-borne illnesses can be found throughout the world. The other less common types include tick-borne and fly-borne arboviral infections. The details of mosquito and other arthropod vectors will be presented in the following chapters. Due to globalization, the change in the epidemiology of illnesses from one place to the other all over the world can be expected. A summative report on the common arboviral illnesses in the tropical and nontropical countries can be and should be carried out. Such a reference can be useful for doctors who, in their current work, do not confront the extraordinary problems of the developing world, but might come face to face with those problems due to the possible migration of illnesses.

Factors Contributing to the Arboviral Infections

Indeed, most arboviral diseases are common in the tropical regions. In addition, many common environmental factors in the tropics relate to arboviral infection. Due to the globalization in the present day, the change in the epidemiology of these arthropod-borne diseases from one site to others all around the world can be expected. Interest in a summative evaluation of the common endemic problems in tropical countries is therefore not limited to doctors presently working in these areas. Similar to general disorders in medicine, two main factors contributing to tropical anemia are inherited and non-inherited factors.

1. Inherited Factor

Host Susceptibility

Host susceptibility is the main underlying factor for many infections. For arboviral infection, Catanzaro et al. noted that modulation of cell surface antigens affected arboviral infection [3]. Because arbovirus infection festors the lytic efficiency of all antibody preparations to the same degree in the cell culture study, Catanzaro et al. suggested some form of host cell antigen re-expression as a mechanism [3]. Lee and Lobigs found that virulence attenuation of the host cell-adapted variants of Murray Valley encephalitis virus was a consequence of their increased dependence on cell surface glycosaminoglycans (GAGs) for attachment and entry [4]. Lee and Lobigs also found that the enhanced affinity of the attenuated variants for GAGs ubiquitously present on cells and extracellular matrices most likely prevented viremia of sufficient magnitude and/or duration required for virus entry into the brain parenchyma [5].

Vector Susceptibility

Vector susceptibility is another point of concern in vector-borne disease. Since the vector is the vehicle for transmission of pathogen, vector susceptibility seems to be important for transportation of pathogen to the host. The relationship between host viremia and vector infection is complex, and there is little experimental information to determine the most accurate model for different arthropod-vector-host systems [6]. Until there is more information, the ability to distinguish the relative importance of different hosts in infecting vectors will remain problematic [6]. There are some interesting research studies on vector susceptibility. Venkatesan et al. reported that spatial and temporal heterogeneity could be observed in *Culex tarsalis* for phenotypic traits including autogeny, virus susceptibility and host preference [7]. Zeidner et al. reported that natural feeding by two arbovirus vectors, *Culex pipiens* and *Aedes aegypti*, had a profound T cell modulatory effect in vivo in virus-susceptible animals, which was not demonstrated in the flavivirus resistant host [8]. Moreover, sialokinin-I and sialokinin-II mimicked the effect of mosquito feeding by modulating the host T cell response [8]. Zeidner et al. noted the potential role of the mosquito vector in potentiating virus transmission in the mammalian host [8].

Susceptibility of Pathogens

Susceptibility of pathogens is important for determining the drug resistance of many pathogens. Similarly, sensitivity of arboviruses to drug such as proteases and cycloheximide is also determined by genetic susceptibility [9-10].

2. Non-inhertied Factor

Sima Zue et al. proposed that, in spite of enormous progress in medical science, the reach of health care in poor, underdeveloped, and tropical countries remained incomplete, uncertain and the probability of the death was still high in these countries [11]. Besides, due to difficult field conditions and limited hospitals in the tropical countries, care is often delayed [11]. As q result, the majority of patients are admitted with the advanced illness and complications [11]. In addition, the local hospital is often poorly equipped, undersupplied and lacks qualified personnel and basic drugs [11]. These situations are also the main concerns regarding tropical arthropod-borne diseases.

Poverty

In other words, poverty carries with it a lack of opportunity to obtain good health and brings many disorders, especially tropical infections, including mosquito-borne tropical illnesses. Lifson recently said that poverty was a factor that contributed to the epidemic of the dengue fever [12]. Other factors that contribute to the epidemic of dengue fever are international travel, urbanization, population growth, a weakened sanitary infrastructure, and limited support for programs to maintain disease control [12]. Pinikahana proposed the need for an investigation to examine whether beliefs and cultural values or poverty prevented some people to utilize bed nets or any other protective device [13]. Therefore, development based on economic growth, to conquer poverty in tropical countries, is necessary and becomes the politic strategy for all developing countries. Development signifies an improvement in quality of life by benefits in health, education, living standards, and increased income [14-15]. The process of urbanization could be described as one of greater, global, and environmental changes directly affecting human health and affecting populations, especially in developing countries, where urban growth, like an express train, has been accompanied by massive urban poverty [14]. One of the adverse effects of development—contamination—has also been proposed as an important factor that applies to arboviral disease in the present.

Poor Hygiene

As previously mentioned, poor hygiene can be the result of poverty. The population—especially the marginal group—in tropical places generally receives poor sanitary services. Mata proposed that the physical environment in the tropics and the socioeconomic characteristics of the population inhabiting such regions favor maintenance and transmission of a variety of viruses, bacteria, and parasites that present roadblocks for agricultural progress and social development [16].

Environmental Temperature and Humidity

Similar to other tropical illnesses, the environmental temperature, generally hot in the tropics, aids in the transmission of many tropical contagious illnesses. There are many investigations on the effect of temperature in arthropod-borne diseases. Besides temperature, humidity is another important factor that affects the spread of the contagious mosquito-borne illness. Humidity mainly affects the breeding of mosquitoes. It should be noted that the frequency of contagious mosquito-borne illnesses in the area of the desert is less common than of area of rain forest.

Pollution

Exposure to environmental contamination remains a main source of health risk throughout the world, although risks are generally higher in developing countries where poverty, lack of the investment in technology and weak environmental legislation combine to cause high levels of contamination [17]. Briggs noted that associations between environmental pollution and health outcome were, nevertheless, complex and often badly characterized [17]. It should be noted that human health cannot remain sustainable if damage to the global environment continues [18]. McMichael proposed a simple argument that "Earth is essentially a closed system; humans are proliferating and commandeering more surface area, food and energy; the resultant accumulation of waste gases, depletion of soil and water, and loss of biodiversity is starting to overload Earth's carrying capacity. There are limits in any closed system and our species is now pressing against some of them. These are new problems and we cannot be certain of the consequences for human health. A warmer world will probably have more frequent heatwaves, unstable weather, increased spread of mosquito-borne infectious diseases, and disruptions to agriculture [18]."

At present, the change in climate is an important factor in the discussion of world health. Epstein noted that computer models predicted that global warming would widen the incidence and distribution of many serious medical disorders [19]. Global warming, aside from indirectly causing death by drowning or starvation, promotes by various means the emergence, resurgence, and, by extension, contagious illnesses [19]. Among the largest health concerns are illnesses transmitted by mosquitoes, such as dengue fever, yellow fever, and several types of encephalitis [19]. Such disorders are projected to come to be increasingly more predominant because the insect vectors are very sensitive to weather conditions [18]. In addition, floods and droughts that result from global warming support each other, as dried insect eggs remains viable when trapped in water [19].

Virology of Arbovirus

As previously mentioned, arbovirus is the name of a group of viruses that can be transmitted via blood-feeding arthropod vectors. Most arboviruses are spherical in shape, although a few are rod shaped. The average size is 17–150 nm in diameter and all have a RNA genome. These RNA viruses do not normally infect humans, but if they do they usually cause several problematic diseases such as dengue infection and yellow fever. Examples of arbovirus are Chikungunya virus, dengue virus, Ross River virus, West Nile virus, yellow fever, Japanese encephalitis virus, La Crosse encephalitis virus, Murray Valley virus, St. Louis Encephalitis virus and O'nyong'nyong virus.

Arboviruses generally require horizontal transmission by arthropod vectors among vertebrate hosts for their natural maintenance [20]. This requirement for alternate replication in disparate hosts places unusual evolutionary constraints on these viruses, which have probably limited the evolution of arboviruses to only a few families of RNA viruses (Togaviridae, Flaviviridae, Bunyaviridae, Rhabdoviridae, Reoviridae, and Orthomyxoviridae) [20]. The three main severe clinical presentations of arbovirus infections are hemorrhagic fever, meningoencephalitis and arthritis. Phylogenetic studies have suggested the dominance of purifying selection in the evolution of arboviruses, consistent with constraints imposed by differing replication environments and requirements in arthropod and vertebrate hosts [20]. Recently, Brown et al. noted that the first demonstration of arbovirus infection increasing with group size was a predictor of an ecological relationship between an arbovirus and its vectors/hosts [21]. In addition, molecular genetic studies of some arboviruses have also identified some mutations that effect differentially the replication in vertebrate and mosquito cells. Weaver et al. found that alternating host transmission cycles could constrain the evolutionary rates of arboviruses but not their fitness for either host alone [22]. These data can help understand the temporal and spatial variation in arboviral epidemics. The mode and tempo of arbovirus evolution and dispersal can help to explain the dynamics of pandemics, viral outbreaks, and emerging viruses [23]. By comparing nucleotide and deduced amino acid sequences of their envelope proteins, the molecular epidemiology change of arboviral infection can be determined [23]. The analyses reveal a correlation between the geographical and genetic distances of these viruses. The arthropod host appears to be a key factor for the formation and maintenance of the dynamic cline [23]. It is confirmed that many pandemics are attributed to the ability of some RNA viruses to change their host range to include humans [24].

Etiologic agents of arboviral diseases are primarily zoonotic pathogens that are maintained in nature in cycles involving arthropod transmission among a variety of susceptible reservoir hosts [25]. In the simplest form of human exposure, spillover occurs from the enzootic cycle when humans enter zoonotic foci and/or enzootic amplification increases circulation near humans; however, two of the most important human arboviral pathogens, yellow fever and dengue viruses, have gone one step further and adopted humans as their amplification hosts, allowing for urban disease [25]. During the past two decades there has been a dramatic resurgence or emergence of epidemic arboviral diseases affecting both humans and domestic animals [26]. These epidemics have been caused primarily by viruses thought to be under control such as dengue, Japanese encephalitis, yellow fever, and

Venezuelan equine encephalitis, or viruses that have expanded their geographic distribution, such as West Nile and Rift Valley fever [26]. Therefore, the emerging and remerging of arboviral infections becomes a new world public health problem. At present, there are over 534 viruses listed in the arbovirus list, approximately 134 of which have been shown to cause disease in humans [27]. Global demographic and societal changes and modern transportation have provided the mechanisms for the viruses to break out of their natural ecology and become established in new geographic locations where susceptible arthropod vectors and hosts provide permissive conditions for them to cause major epidemics [27].

Although the disease manifestations are very diverse, general lessons relevant to optimal use of laboratory resources can be drawn from medically important examples [28]. Standard virology and serology techniques can be used for diagnosis of arboviral infection [29–30]. A classical technique of insect tissue culture is used for arbovirus culture [31–33]. However, this technique is very complicated. Serological diagnosis becomes more widely used. Important considerations for diagnosis include selection of the appropriate clinical specimen, especially for serum and cerebrospinal fluid [34]. At present, arbovirus infection is generally diagnosed serologically. Although none of the newer rapid immunologic techniques is commercially available, some do hold great promise [35]. These include measurement of virus-specific immunoglobulin M (IgM) and detection of viral antigens by enzyme or radioimmunoassay [35]. Recently, the molecular biology technique has helped diagnosis in difficult cases. For example, MacMinn et al. suggested that Murray Valley encephalitis-specific reverse transcriptase-polymerase chain reaction (RT-PCR) provides rapid and specific diagnosis of Murray Valley encephalitis and should be used more widely for the diagnosis of acute viral encephalitis in cases originating from flavivirus endemic areas [36]. According to another study by Ward et al., the PCR technique was found to be as sensitive as a plaque assay for detecting Dugbe (DUG) virus, but not as sensitive as intracerebral inoculation of mice [37]. In this study, the sensitivity of the technique was greatest using crude RNA extracts combined with dot-blot analysis of the resulting PCR products using a DUG-specific cDNA probe, and a result was obtained within 48 h using PCR, whereas biological assays took at least eight days to diagnose the virus infection [37]. Recently, a selected number of PCR protocols were evaluated to determine if they could serve as a universal protocol for detecting and identifying all arboviruses [38]. In this study, four parameters that affect the efficacy of RT-PCR (RNA extraction method, choice of reverse transcriptase, choice of DNA polymerase and thermocycling program) were evaluated in combination [38]. Kuno et al. found that a simultaneous screening of clinical or biological specimens by RT-PCR with the use of a universal diagnostic protocol against a large number of RNA viruses belonging to many families can be performed more efficiently for etiologic determination in the situations complicated by the difficulty of differential diagnosis [38].

Controlling of arboviral diseases can be based on the general principle of controlling for vector-borne diseases. Successful control programs aim at vulnerable points in the interactions between the vector, the reservoir host, the pathogen, the human host, and the environment [39]. The objective is to prevent potential transmission, or interrupt actual transmission, by reducing the abundance, longevity, or host contact of the vector, whichever is most appropriate to the particular pathogen or disease and the local situation [39]. Traditional means of controlling arboviral diseases include vaccination of susceptible vertebrates and mosquito control, but in many cases these have been unavailable or ineffective, and so novel strategies for disease control are needed. Previously successful strategies to control arboviral diseases was vector control, but source reduction and vector control strategies using pesticides have not been sustainable [40]. New insights into vector biology and vector pathogen interactions, and the novel targets that likely will be forthcoming in the vector post-genomics era, provide new targets and opportunities for vector control and disease reduction programs [40]. One new possibility is genetic manipulation of mosquito vectors to render them unable to transmit arboviruses [41]. Of interest, virus-resistant mosquito lines by transformation with transposable elements that express effector RNAs from mosquito-active promoters can be now developed [42]. Advances in vector genomics can offer new promise for the control of arthropod vectors of disease [43]. Hill et al. said that radical changes in vector-biology research were required if scientists are to exploit genomic data and implement changes in public health [43].

New Concerns Regarding Arboviral Infection

A. Terrorism

The causes of the emergence or reemergence of infectious diseases are multiple and diverse, often in direct relation with human activities including population migrations, changes in husbandry or farming practices, worldwide exchanges of goods and foods, and inadequate uses of antibiotics, but also with climatic variations in several areas [44]. Arbovirus infections become emerging or re-emerging diseases that need a multidisciplinary effort to control the propagation of the infectious agent and the pathogenesis in infected patients [45]. Of interest, some viruses could be used for bioterrorism attacks [45]. Many arboviruses that cause hemorrhagic manifestation must be considered dangerous biological weapons that could potentially be used [46]. Most of the viruses responsible for hemorrhagic fever can be transmitted to humans through the air in spray form, except the dengue virus and the agents of hemorrhagic fever from the Congo Crimea and the hemorrhagic fever with renal syndrome that are difficult to handle in cell culture [46].

B. Global Warming Effect

As previously mentioned, environmental factors can contribute to the spreading of arbovirus. Most vector-borne diseases exhibit a distinct seasonal pattern, which clearly suggests that they are weather sensitive [47]. Rainfall, temperature, and other weather variables affect in many ways both the vectors and the pathogens they transmit [47]. For example, high temperatures can increase or reduce survival rate, depending on the vector, its behavior, ecology, and many other factors [47]. Chastel said that global warming [+0.5–0.6°C during the second half of the 20th century] seems a reality, although climatologists have not reached a common agreement on its actual origin, and this phenomenon may still increase during the 21st century [+1.5–6°C] [48]. Particular attention is devoted to the eventual effects of climatic changes on the hibernation process in some small mammals and the timing of birds' migrations involved in enzootic cycles of arboviruses [48]. It is likely that arbovirus diseases may locally extend both in latitude and altitude, leading to outbreaks, but regressions may also occur [48]. Russell said that the predicted scenarios of increased temperature and rainfall with global warming were also causing concern for increases in vector-borne diseases, particularly the endemic arboviruses [49].

C. Travel Medicine and Arboviral Infection

The tremendous growth in international travel increases the risk of importation of vector-borne diseases, some of which can be transmitted locally under suitable circumstances at the right time of the year [47]. Arboviral infection is a focus in travel medicine [50]. There are several case reports of classical arboviral diseases in remote new settings. Thus, with increasing world travel and migration, there is a need for increasing awareness of arboviral infections [51].

References

[1] Vector borne diseases. Available at http://www.fpnotebook.com/ID211.htm

[2] Changes in the Incidence of Vector-Borne Diseases Attributable to Climate Change. Available at http://www.ciesin.org/TG/HH/veclev2.html

[3] Catanzaro PJ, Brandt WE, Hogrefe WR, Phillips SM, Top FH Jr. Virus-enhanced modulation of cell surface antigens: effect on immune lytic susceptibility. *J. Immunol.* 117, 1104-10 (1976)

[4] Lee E, Lobigs M. Substitutions at the putative receptor-binding site of an encephalitic flavivirus alter virulence and host cell tropism and reveal a role for glycosaminoglycans in entry. *J. Virol.* 74, 8867-8875 (2000)

[5] Lee E, Lobigs M. Mechanism of virulence attenuation of glycosaminoglycan-binding variants of Japanese encephalitis virus and Murray Valley encephalitis virus. *J. Virol.* 76, 4901-11 (2002)

[6] Lord CC, Rutledge CR, Tabachnick WJ. Relationships between host viremia and vector susceptibility for arboviruses. *J. Med. Entomol.* 43, 623-30 (2006)

[7] Venkatesan M, Hauer MC, Rasgon JL. Using fluorescently labelled M13-tailed primers to isolate 45 novel microsatellite loci from the arboviral vector Culex tarsalis. *Med. Vet. Entomol.* 21, 204-8 (2007)

[8] Zeidner NS, Higgs S, Happ CM, Beaty BJ, Miller BR. Mosquito feeding modulates Th1 and Th2 cytokines in flavivirus susceptible mice: an effect mimicked by injection of sialokinins, but not demonstrated in flavivirus resistant mice. *Parasite. Immunol.* 21, 35-44. (1999)

[9] Gorman B, Goss P. Sensitivity of arboviruses to proteases. *J. Gen. Virol.* 16:83-6 (1972)

[10] Tonew E, Tonew M. The effect of cycloheximide upon sheep abortion virus, Sindbis virus and other viruses in screening experiments. *Zentralbl. Bakteriol.* [Orig]. 211, 437-44 (1969)

[11] Sima Zue A, Chani M, Ngaka Nsafu D, Carpentier JP. Does tropical environment influence morbidity and mortality? *Med. Trop. (Mars).* 62, 256-9 (2002)

[12] Lifson AR. Mosquitoes, models, and dengue. *Lancet.* 347, 1201-2 (1996)

[13] Pinikahana J. Socio-cultural factors associated with malaria transmission: a review. *Indian J Malariol.* 1992 Jun;29(2):121-6. (1992)

[14] Brinkmann UK. Economic development and tropical disease. *Ann. N. Y. Acad. Sci.* 740, 303-11 (1994)

[15] Stephens C. The urban environment, poverty and health in developing countries. *Health. Policy. Plan.* 10:109-21 (1995)

[16] Mata LJ. The environment of the malnourished child. *Basic. Life. Sci.* 7, 45-66 (1976)

[17] Briggs D. Environmental pollution and the global burden of disease. *Br. Med. Bull.* 68, 1-24 (2003)

[18] McMichael AJ. Global environmental change and human health: new challenges to scientist and policy-maker. *J. Public. Health. Policy.* 15, 407-19 (1994)

[19] Epstein PR. Is global warming harmful to health? *Sci. Am.* 283, 50-7 (2000)

[20] Weaver SC. Evolutionary influences in arboviral disease. *Curr. Top. Microbiol. Immunol.* 299, 285-314 (2006)

[21] Brown CR, Komar N, Quick SB, Sethi RA, Panella NA, Brown MB, Pfeffer M. Arbovirus infection increases with group size. *Proc. Biol. Sci.* 268, 1833-40 (2001)

[22] Weaver SC, Brault AC, Kang W, Holland JJ. Genetic and fitness changes accompanying adaptation of an arbovirus to vertebrate and invertebrate cells. *J. Virol.* 73, 4316-26 (1999)

[23] Zanotto PM, Gao GF, Gritsun T, Marin MS, Jiang WR, Venugopal K, Reid HW, Gould EA. An arbovirus cline across the northern hemisphere. *Virology.* 210,152-9 (1995)

[24] Weaver SC, Barrett AD. Transmission cycles, host range, evolution and emergence of arboviral disease. *Nat. Rev. Microbiol.* 2, 789-801 (2004)

[25] Weaver SC. Host range, amplification and arboviral disease emergence. *Arch. Virol. Suppl.* 19, 33-44 (2005)

[26] Gubler DJ. The global emergence/resurgence of arboviral diseases as public health problems. *Arch. Med.Res.* 33, 330-42 (2002)

[27] Gluber DJ. Human arbovirus infections worldwide. *Ann. N. Y. Acad. Sci.* 951, 13-24 (2001)

[28] Grimley PM. The laboratory role in diagnosis of infections transmitted by arthropods. *Clin. Lab. Med.* 21, 495-512, viii (2001)

[29] Niklasson B. Arbovirus diseases—a review. *Lakartidningen.* 1947-8 (1987)

[30] Draganescu N. Laboratory diagnosis of arbovirus infections. *Stud. Cercet. Inframicrobiol.* 17, 153-65 (1966)

[31] Hink WF. Insect tissue culture. *Adv. Appl. Microbiol.* 15, 157-214 (1972)

[32] Singh KR. Growth of arboviruses in arthropod tissue culture. *Adv. Virus. Res.* 17, 187-206 (1972)

[33] Yunker CE. Arthropod tissue culture in the study of arboviruses and rickettsiae: a review. *Curr. Top. Microbiol. Immunol.* 55, 113-26 (1971)

[34] Bloch KC, Glaser C.Diagnostic approaches for patients with suspected encephalitis. *Curr. Infect. Dis. Rep.* 9, 315-22 (2007)

[35] Rubin RJ. Detection of viruses in spinal fluid. *Am. J. Med.* 75, 124-8 (1983)

[36] McMinn PC, Carman PG, Smith DW. Early diagnosis of Murray Valley encephalitis by reverse transcriptase-polymerase chain reaction. *Pathology.* 32, 49-51 (2000)

[37] Ward VK, Marriott AC, Booth TF, el-Ghorr AA, Nuttall PA. Detection of an arbovirus in an invertebrate and a vertebrate host using the polymerase chain reaction. *J. Virol. Methods.* 30, 291-300 (1990)

[38] Kuno G. Universal diagnostic RT-PCR protocol for arboviruses. *J. Virol. Methods.* 72, 27-41 (1998)

[39] Russell RC. Vector-borne diseases and their control. *Med. J. Aust.* 158, 681, 684-90 (1993)

[40] Beaty BJ. Control of arbovirus diseases: is the vector the weak link? *Arch. Virol. Suppl.* 19, 73-88 (2005)

[41] Blair CD, Adelman ZN, Olson KE. Molecular strategies for interrupting arthropod-borne virus transmission by mosquitoes. *Clin. Microbiol. Rev.* 13, 651-61 (2000)

[42] Olson KE, Adelman ZN, Travanty EA, Sanchez-Vargas I, Beaty BJ, Blair CD. Developing arbovirus resistance in mosquitoes. *Insect. Biochem. Mol. Biol.* 32, 1333-43 (2002)

[43] Hill CA, Kafatos FC, Stansfield SK, Collins FH. Arthropod-borne diseases: vector control in the genomics era. *Nat. Rev. Microbiol.* 3, 262-8 (2005)

[44] Werner GH. The worldwide challenges of "new" or reemerging communicable diseases at the dawn of the 21st century. *Ann. Pharm. Fr.* 59, 246-77 (2001)

[45] Deubel V, Georges-Courbot MC. Arboviruses and epizootic viruses. *C. R. Biol.* 325, 855-61; 879-83 (2002)

[46] Rigaudeau S, Bricaire F, Bossi P. Haemorrhagic fever viruses, possible bioterrorist use. *Presse. Med.* 34, 169-76 (2005)

[47] Gubler DJ, Reiter P, Ebi KL, Yap W, Nasci R, Patz JA. Climate variability and change in the United States: potential impacts on vector- and rodent-borne diseases. *Environ. Health. Perspect.* 109 Suppl 2, 223-33 (2001)

[48] Chastel C. Impact of global climate changes on arboviruses transmitted to humans by mosquitoes and ticks. *Bull. Acad. Natl. Med.* 186, 89-100; 100-1 (2002)

[49] Russell RC. Vectors vs. humans in Australia—who is on top down under? An update on vector-borne disease and research on vectors in Australia. *J. Vector. Ecol.* 23, 1-46 (1998)

[50] Wolfe MS. Travel medicine. *Curr. Opin. Infect. Dis.* 12, 433-8 (1999)

[51] Abebajo AO. Rheumatic manifestations of tropical diseases. *Curr. Opin. Rheumatol.* 8, 85-9 (1996)

Chapter I

Non-Mosquito Arbovirus Vector

Introduction to Arthropod Vector and Medical Entomology

Arthropod-borne infection is an important group of infectious diseases. The arthropod, a many jointed-leg animal, is the main vector for arthropod-borne infection. Indeed, the arthropod can be seen everywhere all over the world. Transmission of arbovirus is based on the principle of the epidemiological triad: host, pathogen and environment. Among animal viruses, arboviruses are unique in that they depend on arthropod vectors for transmission [1]. Field research and laboratory investigations related to the three components of this unique mode of transmission—virus, vector, and vertebrate host—have produced an enormous amount of valuable information that may be found in numerous publications [1]. Diseases that are transmitted by arthropods cause severe morbidity and mortality throughout the world [2]. The burden of many of these diseases is borne largely by developing countries [2]. Blood- sucking insects are the vectors of arboviruses. Basically, animal skin separates the inner world of the body from the largely hostile outside world and is actively involved in the defense against microbes [3]. However, the skin is not a perfect defence barrier and many microorganisms have managed to live on or within the skin as harmless passengers or as disease-causing pathogens [3]. A number of pathogens use arthropod vectors, like ticks or mosquitoes, to deliver them into the dermis while taking their blood meal [3]. Within the dermis, successful pathogens subvert the function of a variety of skin resident cells or cells of the innate immune system that rush to the site of infection [3].

Study of the arthropod is the main section of medical entomology. Medical entomology is the basic field of knowledge for the general practitioner in the diagnosis and treatment of arthropod-borne disease. A new concept of medical entomology is proposed, according to which this discipline should comprehensively study the effects of arthropods on human health and possible control of these effects [4]. The recent biotechnological revolution in molecular entomology explores new promising tools for the control of vector-borne diseases through genetic manipulation of vectorial competence [5]. At present, the most common arthropod vector for arboviral infections is the mosquito. The details on medically-important mosquitoes will be presented in the next chapter. In this chapter, the details on non-mosquito arbovirus vectors will be presented.

Medically Important Tick Vectors for Arbovirus

Ticks are the second most common arboviral vectors. Ticks are small wingless bloodsucking insects. Indeed, ticks can transmit many diseases in additional to arbovirus infections. It has been known for many years that tick-borne diseases have worldwide a high economical impact on the farming industry and veterinary medicine [4]. But only in the last twenty years has the importance of such diseases been recognized in human medicine by the medical community and the public with emergence of the tick-borne encephalitis virus and the description of *Borrelia burgdorferi* [5]. The details of medically-important ticks that cause arthropod-borne arboviral infection are hereby presented.

1. *Dermacentor* Species

The Rocky Mountain wood tick, *Dermacentor andersoni*, is the primary vector for Colorado tick fever, a well-known tick-borne arboviral infection [6]. Seasonal activity and Colorado tick fever virus infection rates in Rocky Mountain wood ticks, *Dermacentor andersoni,* is well described [8]. The morphology of *Dermacentor andersoni* was first described by Stiles in 1908. The anus is located in the median line, posterior to the last pair of legs. Of interest, a single adult male *Dermacentor andersoni* Rocky Mountain wood tick was collected that exhibited unique morphological anomalies, including the absence of a leg on the right side of the body [9]. Coxa IV on the right side also was missing in this specimen. This is an interesting report on abnormal morphology of *Dermacentor andersoni* [9]. Restricted in habitat to the Rocky Mountains in the United States and southwestern Canada, the Rocky Mountain wood tick's life cycle may require between two and three years for completion [10]. Although adult ticks feed primarily on large mammals including humans, the larval and nymph forms feast on small rodents [10]. Similar to most tick species, *Dermacentor andersoni* requires a blood meal before developing into its next life stage [10]. In addition to *Dermacentor andersoni*, there are also some other important species. *Dermacentor reticulatus* is an example that can cause babesiosis [11]. It should be noted that many tick-borne diseases are endemic, in particular the way in which main carrier ticks prefer, for their vital cycle, climatic conditions characterized by high temperatures and a warmth-humid atmosphere [12].

2. *Ixodes* Species

Ixodes ricinus is an important tick that can cause tick-borne arboviral infection. Tick-borne encephalitis is an important disease caused by *Ixodes ricinus*. Tick-borne encephalitis (TBE) virus as a typical arbovirus relies on two types of hosts for its survival: ticks act both as virus vectors and reservoir hosts, and vertebrates amplify the virus infection by acting as a source of infection for feeding ticks [13]. TBE is the major European arbovirosis. In addition to *Ixodes ricinus* in general areas of Europe, *Ixodes persulcatus* is mentioned as the main vector in the Far-Eastern Soviet Union [14]. These ticks are characterized by a comparatively long life cycle, lasting several years, during which the infecting virus may be maintained from one developmental stage of the tick to the next [15-17]. Rodgers et al. reported that ticks did not survive when exposed to dry air for long periods; however, the return of humid air within four to eight hours had as large a positive impact on tick survival as does constant humid air [18]. Korotkov et al. reported that the metamorphosis of tick-borne encephalitis virus-induced *Ixodes ricinus* nymphs under long-day photoperiodic conditions (18 light hours and 6 darkness hours) occured more rapidly than in uninfected specimens [19]. In addition to arbovirus, *Ixodes ricinus* is also an important vector for rickettsia. Lyme disease is an important example of rickettsial infection related to this tick. The field and laboratory evidence incriminating nymphal *Ixodes ricinus* as an important vector of *Borrelia burgdorferi*, the causative pathogen of Lyme disease, is substantial [20].

3. *Ornithodoros* Species

African swine fever virus (ASFV) is the only known DNA arbovirus and the sole member of the family *Asfarviridae*. It causes a lethal, hemorrhagic disease in domestic pigs. ASFV is enzootic in sub-Saharan Africa and is maintained in a sylvatic cycle by infecting both wild members of the *Suidae* and the argasid tick *Ornithodoros porcinus porcinus* [21]. The mechanism of ASFV transmission from the sylvatic cycle to domestic pigs is probably through infected ticks feeding on pigs [22]. In addition to *Ornithodoros porcinus porcinus*, a number of North American, Central American and Caribbean species of *Ornithodoros* have been shown to be potential vectors of ASFV [22]. Kleiboeker et al. indicated that virus replication was restricted in midgut epithelial cells of *Ornithodoros porcinus porcinus* [23]. This finding demonstrates the importance of viral replication in the midgut for successful ASFV infection of the arthropod host [23].

Medically Important Fly Vectors for Arbovirus

There are many flies throughout the world. However, there are only a few species that can act as vectors of diseases. The details of medically-important flies that cause arthropod-borne arboviral infection are hereby presented.

1. *Phlcbotomus* Species

Sandfly fever is an important arboviral infection. *Phlebotomus* species is the main vector for sandfly fever. *Phlebotomus perniciosus* is the main vector species. Concerning the morphology of *Phlebotomus* species, during larval development, thoracic and abdominal spiracles show considerable modifications [24]. In fourth instar larvae, the spiracles consist of a plate with a sclerotized central portion and a peripheral circle of papillae [24]. Fausto et al. reported that the seminal vesicles of *Phlebotomus perniciosus* had a complex structure, and three different morphological compartments, called A, B and C [25]. Compartment A is continuous with the vasa deferentia and consists of a cylindrical wall limiting a lumen in which the spermatozoa are stored [25]. Compartment B is hemispherical and surrounds compartment A like a muff [25]. Compartment C constitutes an external coat surrounding A and B [25]. Fausto et al. reported that the epithelial cells of each compartment are characterized by morphologically different secretory granules [25]. Benito-De Martin studied influence of the nature of the ingested blood on the gonotrophic parameters of *Phlebotomus perniciosus* under laboratory conditions [26]. They found that the pre-oviposition and egg incubation periods were not affected whatever the blood ingested by the female. In addition to sandfly fever, *Phlebotomus* species is also the vector of the well known blood infection, leishmaniasis.

2. *Simulium* Species

Simulium vittatum females are shown to be competent vectors for the New Jersey serotype (VSNJ) of vesicular stomatitis virus (Camp Verde strain) [27]. In 1992, Cupp et al. first found that this black fly played a major role in the epizootic transmission of VSNJ. Cupp et al. noted in their report that "This is also the first confirmed example of biological transmission of an arbovirus by a member of the *Simuliidae*" [27]. In 1999, Mead et al. demonstrated that black flies were involved in VSV-NJ transmission during epizootics in the western United States and represent the first confirmed example of biological transmission of an arbovirus by a member of the *Simuliidae* using an animal model [28]. In the black flies, salivary gland involvement of virus is more likely [29]. However, Howerth et al. suggested a more generalized infection that apparently circumvented the gut as evidenced in their viral staining studies [29]. According to their study, extensive staining of eye, brain, and hemolymph could also be seen [29].

References

[1] Kuno G, Chang GJ. Biological transmission of arboviruses: reexamination of and new insights into components, mechanisms, and unique traits as well as their evolutionary trends. *Clin. Microbiol. Rev.* 18, 608-37 (2005)

[2] Hill CA, Kafatos FC, Stansfield SK, Collins FH. Arthropod-borne diseases: vector control in the genomics era. *Nat. Rev. Microbiol.* 3, 262-8 (2005)

[3] Frischknecht F. The skin as interface in the transmission of arthropod-borne pathogens. *Cell. Microbiol.* 9, 1630-40 (2007)

[4] Rasnitsyn SP. The concept of medical entomology: the determination of the effect of arthropods on human health. *Izv. Akad. Nauk. Ser. Biol.* 4, 437-45 (1996)

[5] Joardar GK. Molecular entomology: a new promising tool for malaria control. *Indian. J. Public. Health.* 49, 231-4 (2005)

[6] Wahlberg P, Carlsson SA, Granlund H, Jansson C, Linden M, Nyberg C, Nyman D. Holzer BR. Tick borne diseases. *Ther. Umsch.* 62, 757-63 (2005)

[7] Klasco R. Colorado tick fever. *Med. Clin. North. Am.* 86, 435-40 (2002)

[8] Eads RB, Smith GC. Seasonal activity and Colorado tick fever virus infection rates in Rocky Mountain wood ticks, Dermacentor andersoni (acari: Ixodidae), in north-central Colorado, USA. *J. Med. Entomol.* 20, 49-55 (1983)

[9] Dergousoff SJ, Chilton NB. Abnormal morphology of an adult Rocky Mountain wood tick, Dermacentor andersoni (Acari: Ixodidae). *J. Parasitol.* 93, 708-9 (2007)

[10] Kelly CD, Fellers TJ, Davidson MW. Rocky Mountain Wood Tick. Available online at http://72.14.235.104/search?q=cache:kYJZRRr6mbgJ:www.olympusmicro.com/micd/galleries/oblique/rockymountainwoodtick.html

[11] Heile C, Heydorn AO, Schein E. Dermacentor reticulatus (Fabricius, 1794)--distribution, biology and vector for Babesia canis in Germany. *Berl. Munch. Tierarztl. Wochenschr.* 119, 330-4 (2006)

[12] Torina A, Caracappa S. Dog tick-borne diseases in Sicily. *Parassitologia.* 48, 145-7 (2006)

[13] Labuda M, Eleckova E, Lickova M, Sabo A. Tick-borne encephalitis virus foci in Slovakia. *Int. J. Med. Microbiol.* 291 Suppl 33, 43-7 (2002)

[14] Hannoun C. Tick-borne encephalitis in Europe (author's transl). *Med. Trop. (Mars).* 40, 509-19 (1980)

[15] Pogodina VV. Monitoring of tick-borne encephalitis virus populations and etiological structure of morbidity over 60 years. *Vopr. Virusol.* 50, 7-13 (2005)

[16] Rizzoli A, Rosa R, Mantelli B, Pecchioli E, Hauffe H, Tagliapietra V, Beninati T, Neteler M, Genchi C. Ixodes ricinus, transmitted diseases and reservoirs. *Parassitologia.* 46, 119-22 (2004)

[17] Nuttall PA, Labuda M. Dynamics of infection in tick vectors and at the tick-host interface. *Adv. Virus. Res.* 60, 233-72 (2003)

[18] Rodgers SE, Zolnik CP, Mather TN. Duration of exposure to suboptimal atmospheric moisture affects nymphal blacklegged tick survival. *J. Med. Entomol.* 44, 372-5 (2007)

[19] Korotkov IuS, Burenkova LA, Pivanova GP. Tick-borne encephalitis virus as an amplifier of the metamorphosis of Ixodes ricinus (Acari: Ixodidae) tick nymphs under long-day photoperiodic conditions. *Med. Parazitol. (Mosk).* 4, 52-5 (2006)

[20] Piesman J. Transmission of Lyme disease spirochetes (Borrelia burgdorferi). *Exp. Appl. Acarol.* 7, 71-80 (1989)

[21] Kleiboeker SB, Scoles GA. Pathogenesis of African swine fever virus in Ornithodoros ticks. *Anim. Health. Res. Rev.* 2, 121-8 (2001)

[22] Kleiboeker SB, Scoles GA. Pathogenesis of African swine fever virus in Ornithodoros ticks. *Anim. Health. Res. Rev* 2, 121-8 (2001)

[23] Kleiboeker SB, Scoles GA, Burrage TG, Sur J. African swine fever virus replication in the midgut epithelium is required for infection of Ornithodoros ticks. *J. Virol.* 73, 8587-98 (1999)

[24] Fausto AM, Taddei AR, Mazzini M, Maroli M. Morphology and ultrastructure of spiracles in phlebotomine sandfly larvae. *Med. Vet. Entomol.* 13, 101-9 (1999)

[25] Fausto AM, Gambellini G, Taddei AR, Maroli M, Mazzini M. Ultrastructure of the seminal vesicle of Phlebotomus perniciosus Newstead (Diptera, Psychodidae). *Tissue. Cell.* 32, 228-37 (2000)

[26] Benito-De Martin MI, Gracia-Salinas MJ, Molina-Moreno R, Ferrer-Dufol M, Lucientes-Curdi J. Influence of the nature of the ingested blood on the gonotrophic parameters of Phlebotomus perniciosus under laboratory conditions. *Parasite.* 1, 409-11 (1994)

[27] Cupp EW, Mare CJ, Cupp MS, Ramberg FB. Biological transmission of vesicular stomatitis virus (New Jersey) by Simulium vittatum (Diptera: Simuliidae). *J. Med. Entomol.* 29, 137-40 (1992)

[28] Mead DG, Mare CJ, Ramberg FB. Bite transmission of vesicular stomatitis virus (New Jersey serotype) to laboratory mice by Simulium vittatum (Diptera: Simuliidae). *J. Med. Entomol.* 36, 410-3 (1999)

[29] Howerth EW, Mead DG, Stallknecht DE. Immunolocalization of vesicular stomatitis virus in black flies (Simulium vittatum). *Ann. N. Y. Acad. Sci.* 969, 340-5 (2002)

Chapter II

Medically Important Mosquitoes

What Is a "Mosquito"?

The mosquito is a well-known insect. Based on taxonomy, the mosquito is a eukaryote, the domain that contains all of the organisms whose cells have a nucleus and other membrane-bound bodies [1]. In eukaryota, the mosquito is categorized as a metazoan, the category that includes all of the animals [1]. Mosquitoes are members of the phylum Arthropoda, the largest phylum of all animals [1]. Within the arthropods, the mosquito is a member in the class Insecta [1–2]. It specifically belongs to the order Diptera, which are true flies [1]. Briefly, the Diptera derive their name from the fact that they only have two functional wings, the second pair having been reduced to "halters," or lost altogether (Figure 1) [2]. In Diptera, the mosquito is classified into the suborder Nematocera, family Culicidae, and subfamily Culicinae. Concerning the life cycle of a mosquito, all mosquitoes have four stages of development—egg, larva, pupa, and adult—and they spend their larval and pupal stages in water [1–2] (Figure 2).

Usually, female mosquitoes deposit their eggs (Figure 3, Figure 4) on moist surfaces that may be near water but dry, such as mud or fallen leaves; however, at a later time, rain or high tides typically flood these surfaces and stimulate the eggs to hatch into larvae [3]. The females of other species deposit their eggs directly on the surface of still water in such places as ditches, abandoned containers, streams that are drying up, and fields or excavations that hold water for some time [3]. Dieng et al. noted that larvae of the mosquito *Aedes* species typically develop in small aquatic sites such as tree holes and artificial containers [4]. They noted that organic detritus—in particular, decaying leaves—is, therefore, their major carbon source [4]. Dieng et al. demonstrated the importance of leaf characteristics and, in particular, rates of decay, in determining the development and survivorship of larvae by comparing the effects of a rapidly decaying leaf, the maple *Acer buergerianum* and a slowly decaying leaf, the camphor *Cinnamomum japonicum*, on the larval development of *Aedes albopictus* at different larval densities in laboratory microcosms [4]. According to this study, the maple leaves provided a better substrate and the observed growth patterns could be explained on the basis of a difference in nutritive and chemical contents of the two leaf types [4].

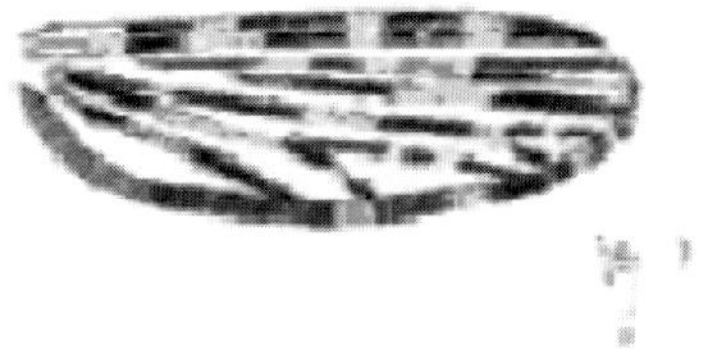

Wiwanitkit V, 2005.
* The mosquito wing in this picture is of Anopheline group.

Figure 1. Drawing of a mosquito wing.

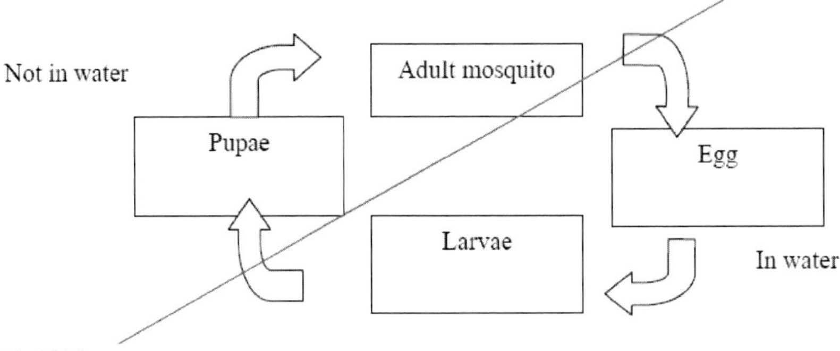

Wiwanitkit V, 2005.

Figure 2. Life cycle of a mosquito

Dieng et al. found that rapidly decaying leaf litter favors mosquito growth, resulting in quicker development and higher population sizes [4]. In conclusion, Dieng et al. emphasized the importance of the local environment on the development of vector mosquitoes and the implications for control [4].

Indeed, many water sources are often stagnant and close to the home in ornamental pools, unused wading and swimming pools, abandoned containers, uncapped jars, animal baths, plant saucers, and even gutters and flat roofs. Mosquito eggs deposited on the surface of such contained water soon hatch into larvae [3]. To control the mosquito, it is necessary to control these water sources. Control of water sources close to the home is widely mentioned, especially for control of dengue. Surveillance of the larvae in water containers is a part of the surveillance of dengue infection. In 2002, population densities of *Aedes aegypti* in four towns in Trinidad were studied using standard house-to-house inspections of all water-holding containers to determine whether persistently positive containers and premises existed over a three-month period in the wet season [5]. According to this study, a total of 24,439 containers were inspected and 1.3% was positive for *Aedes aegypti* larvae and pupae [5]. A total of 16,507 immature *Aedes aegypti* were retrieved from these containers which comprised 17 container types, but when these were ranked according to productivity levels, only water drums (53.5%), buckets (22.2%), tubs and basins (8.0%), water tanks (5.4%), brick holes (4.2%), and tires (2.0%) were significant producers of mosquito larvae [5]. Chadee suggested that *Aedes aegypti* control programs could be more cost effective and sustainable by concentrating efforts on key premises and key containers in order to control mosquito densities and dengue transmission while reducing manpower needs and insecticide use [5].

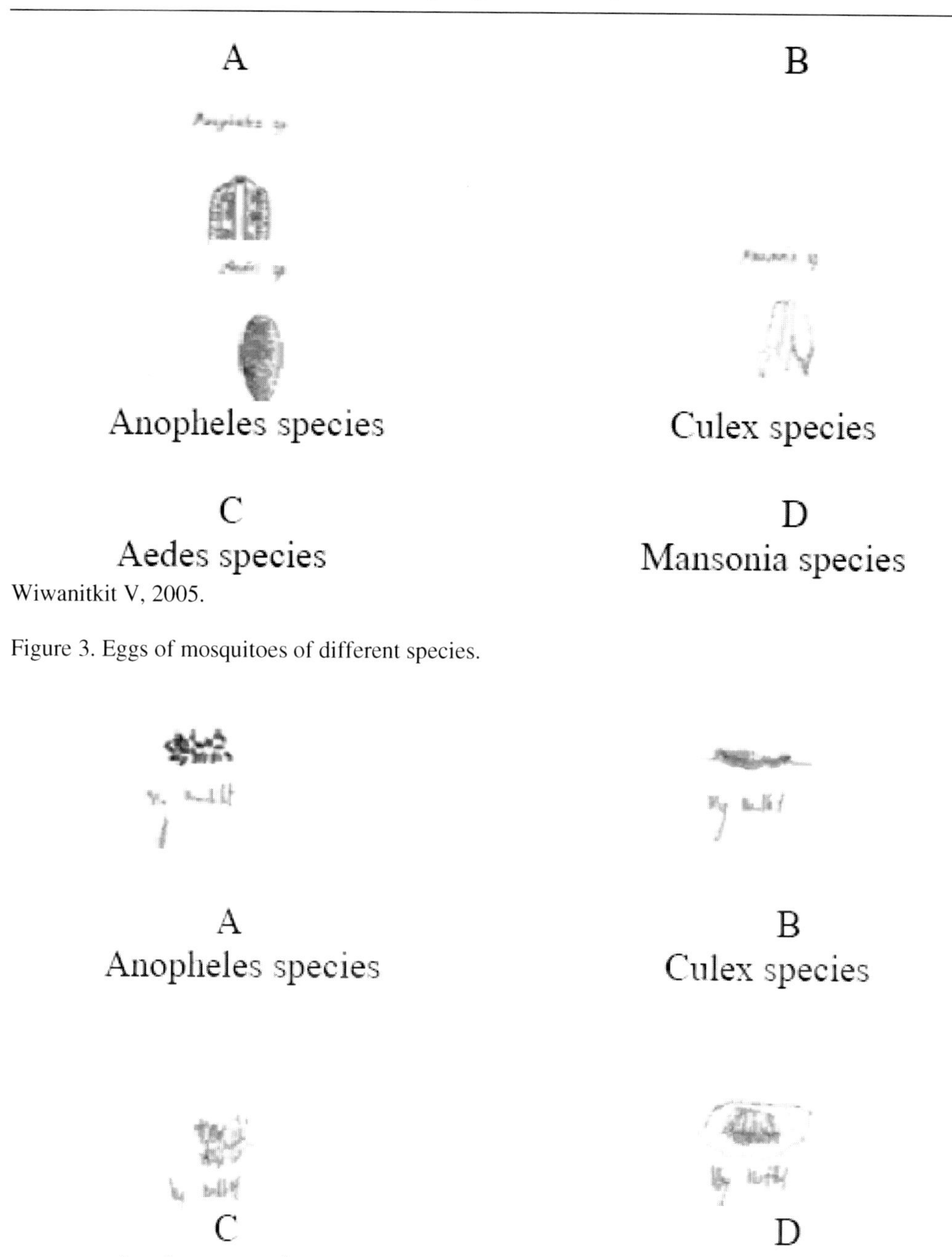

Figure 3. Eggs of mosquitoes of different species.

Figure 4. Arrangement of groups of eggs of mosquitoes of different species.

In the hot summer months, larvae grow rapidly, become pupae, and emerge later as flying adult mosquitoes. In 2002, Lounibos et al. compared growth and survivorship of the two mosquito species, *Aedes aegypti* and *Aedes albopictus,* at controlled temperatures of 24° and 30° C in water-containing tires under conditions of intra- and inter-specific competition, both with and without leaf litter [6]. According to this study, when other variables were controlled statistically, the estimated finite rate of increase (i.e., lambda) was significantly higher for both species at the higher temperature, and the proportional increases in lambda did not differ between species [6]. Lounibos et al. proposed that temperatures between 24° and 30° C would not alter the outcome of larval competition. However, response measures of *Aedes albopictus* were more sensitive than those of *Aedes aegypti* to the litter and species/density variables [6]. In tropical countries, adult mosquitoes usually appear in the early part of the rainy season. The seasonal variation of a mosquito vector is noted. Recently, Wiwanitkit and Suyaphan noted an interesting decrease in the malarial mosquito vector during the summer in a rural community in northern Thailand [7]. Shililu et al. recently conducted entomological studies over a 24-month period in eight villages in order to establish behavior patterns, seasonal densities, and variation in entomological inoculation rates (EIRs) of *Anopheles arabiensis*, the main vector of malaria in Eritrea [8]. They found that population density increased during the rainy season [8]. Conclusively, most mosquitoes spend their adult life during the rainy season, not the summer. Indeed, adult mosquito populations fluctuate and are forced by many variables, especially rainfall, temperature, and humidity. In 2004, Edillo et al. observed the survivorship and distribution of larvae and pupae of *Anopheles gambiae* immature stages in three habitats (rock pools, swamps, and puddles) in Banambani village, Mali, West Africa. During the mid-rainy season, they found that there were obviously unstable age distributions in swamps and puddles and, to some extent, in rock pools; there were also more individuals in some later age classes than in earlier ones [9]. Edillo et al. also noted daily survival estimates using an exponential decay model of 0.807 in rock pools, 0.899 in swamps, 0.818 in puddles, and 0.863 in the overall village [9].

Considering the life cycle of a mosquito, when an adult emerges from the aquatic stage, it mates and the female seeks a blood meal to obtain the protein necessary for the development of her eggs, while the male mosquito does not take a blood meal but may feed on plant nectar [3]. It is important to recognize that young adult female mosquitoes taking their first blood meal do not transmit diseases because they have not yet acquired pathogens that they can spread [3]. While sucking a blood meal, the female mosquito may also inoculate a pathogen into their prey. Shililu et al. reported that annual EIRs varied greatly depending on the year [10]. They noted that EIR profiles indicate that the risk of exposure to infected mosquitoes is highly heterogeneous and seasonal, with high inoculation rates during the rainy season, and little or no transmission during the dry season [10]. Shililu et al. proposed the need to generate spatial and temporal data on transmission intensity on smaller scales to guide targeted control of mosquito-borne disease [10]. In 2005, Nirmala et al. studied the accumulation of specific mitochondrial RNAs (mRNAs) following multiple blood meals in *Anopheles gambiae* [11]. In this study, the mRNA accumulation profiles of eight different genes expressed specifically in the midgut, salivary glands, and body fat tissues of the malarial vector, *Anopheles gambiae*, were characterized as a measure of their suitability to direct the expression of effectors designed to disable specific stages of the parasites [11]. Nirmala et al. found that the multiple feeding behavior of *Anopheles gambiae* could be an advantage in expressing high levels of anti-parasite effectors in order to counteract the parasites throughout most of their adult development stage [11]. Dana et al. said that blood feeding, or hematophagy, was a behavior exhibited by female mosquitoes that is required both for reproduction and for transmission of pathogens [12]. In 2005, Dana et al. determined the expression patterns of 3068 ESTs, representing approximately 2000 unique gene transcripts using complementary DNA (cDNA) microarrays in adult female *Anopheles gambiae* at selected times during the first two days following blood ingestion. At 5 and 30 minutes during a 40-minute blood meal, and at 0, 1, 3, 5, 12, 16, 24 and 48 hours after completion of the blood meal, their expression to transcript levels were compared to mosquitoes with access only to a sugar solution [12]. According to this study, 413 unique transcripts (i.e., approximately 25% of the total) were expressed at least two-fold above or below the levels in the sugar-fed mosquitoes at one or more time points. These differentially expressed gene products were clustered using k-means clustering into early genes, middle genes, and late genes, containing 144, 130, and 139 unique transcripts, respectively [12]. Smith et al. reported that the human biting rate was highest shortly after mosquito densities peak, near breeding sites where adult mosquitoes emerge, and around the edges of areas where humans aggregate [13]. They also noted that the proportion of mosquitoes that were infectious reflected the age structure of the mosquito populations, which peaked where old mosquitoes were found, far from mosquito breeding habitat, and when mosquito population density was declining [13]. Finally, Smith et al. proposed that estimates for the average risk of infection that are based on the average EIR are strongly biased in heterogeneous environments [13].

2. The Role of the Mosquito in Medical Entomology

A. Mosquito-borne Disease

Mosquito-borne disease is a focused area in medical entomology at present. Many mosquito-borne diseases are endemic to tropical areas and become new, emerging infectious diseases in non-endemic areas. Changes in the world environment, globalization, and easily accessed transportation systems are widely mentioned as important factors for changing the present pattern of mosquito-borne infectious diseases. The details of each important mosquito-borne disease will be presented in the following chapters. Mouchet and Bellec said that improved technologies in molecular biology and genetics, supported by computer use, have brought about considerable advances in taxonomy, physiology, host/parasite relationships, ecology, and epidemiology [14]. Alekseev emphasized that medical entomology as a science could not develop, since man-made changes of the environment abound and predicted global warming of the Earth's climate has not been taken into account; indeed, the present status of medical entomological service is considered to be poor [15]. Alekseev noted that the major problems facing medical entomology as a science and the practicality of health care facilities have allowed an outline of tasks to be solved in order of their priority and significance, including the study and monitoring of many mosquito-borne infections, especially the resurgence of malaria [15]. Chow stated that resurgent interest and need was created to promote and support medical entomology [16]. Chow noted that steps should be taken to strengthen the training of workers in medical entomology, to establish a society for vector ecology and control, to issue periodicals, and to coordinate with foreign institutions [16]. Lehane said that the continuing need for vector control in campaigns against insect-transmitted disease is shown by reference to current control programs mounted against several mosquito-borne diseases such as lymphatic filariasis [17].

Control of mosquito-borne infectious diseases is an important issue in public health care. Concerning mosquito control, Mulla noted that vector control technology at first was relatively simple and utilized source reduction, larvivorous fish, petroleum hydrocarbon oils, and some simple synthetic and botanical materials. Then, various classes of synthetic organic chemicals, improved petroleum oil formulations, insect growth regulators, synthetic pyrethroids, and microbial control agents were developed and employed in mosquito control as well as in the control of other disease-vectoring insects [18]. Mouchet and Bellec reported that new insecticides and bacteria are available [14]. Curtis said that there are social, economic, and entomological problems with conventional insecticidal spraying methods for vector control; therefore, there is interest in alternative technologies, especially the impregnation of bed nets with pyrethroid insecticides against mosquito vectors [19]. Curtis said that the bed net method is cheap, socially acceptable, and effective where bed nets are already widely used and where malarial transmission is not very intense; however, in holoendemic areas and where people consider bed nets unaffordable, there are still unanswered questions [19]. Curtis noted that the issue of whether pyrethroid resistance would be selected in *anophelines* also deserves more attention than it has so far attracted, and the application of floating layers of polystyrene beads is a long-lasting and effective control method for Culex mosquitoes [19]. Mouchet and Bellec noted that both simple methods, such as impregnated bed nets and large programs using heavy material have been successful [14]. They noted that mosquito control still has difficulties and needs new tools and a better use of those tools that already exist [14]. Lehane said that successful campaigns have not been reliant on new breakthroughs but on the forging of available tools into effective strategies widely and efficiently used by the control authorities, and the long-lasting political commitment to the success of the schemes in question [17]. Lehane also mentioned that great care is need by policy makers in order to achieve a balance between long-term research that aims at the production of fundamentally new control technologies and operational research aiming to forge the often highly effective tools we already have, into sound control strategies [17]. Mouchet and Bellec concluded that appropriate structures, well-trained and motivated personnel, adequate funding, and political willingness were the keys for the implementation of any control programs [14]. More details on mosquito control and prevention are presented in the final chapter of this book.

B. Mosquito Allergy

Adverse reactions to mosquito bites have been recognized for many years. Peng and Simons said that reactions to mosquito bites were immunological in nature, with the involvement of IgE-, IgG-, and T lymphocyte-mediated hypersensitivities [20]. In addition to local allergic reaction to an itching lesion, there are also other reactions, including large local swellings and redness, generalized urticaria, and angioedema as well as less easily definable responses such as nausea, dizziness, headaches, and lethargy [21]. Reunala et al. said that systemic reactions to mosquito bites were, however, very rare [22]. Peng and Simons noted that an acquired desensitization to mosquito saliva might occur during childhood and adolescence or during long-term exposure to mosquito bites [20]. Reunala et al. said that most people were sensitized to mosquito bites in childhood, and cutaneous symptoms include immediate wheal-and-flare reactions and delayed bite papules, which tend to be more severe at the onset of the mosquito season [22]. Recent immunoblot studies confirm that specific sensitization occurs in man and indicates that mosquito-bite whealing is a classic type I allergic reaction. The delayed mosquito-bite papules seem to be cutaneous late-phase reactions mediated by eosinophils, or they could also represent type IV lymphocyte-mediated immune reactions [22]. Peng and Simons proposed that allergic reactions to mosquito bites are underdiagnosed and undertreated due to the lack of salivary preparations [20]. McCormack et al. reported that two patients experienced systemic anaphylaxis from mosquito bites [21]. In this report, both patients were skin tested and given immunotherapy using whole body mosquito extracts, and it was found that skin testing using whole body mosquito extracts was positive to *Aedes aegypti* at 1/1000 weight/volume (wt/vol) in one patient, *Aedes aegypti* at 1/100,000 wt/vol, and *Culex pipiens* at 1/10,000 wt/vol in the other patient [21]. McCormack et al. reported that immunotherapy using these extracts resulted in resolution of adverse reactions to mosquito bites in one patient and a decrease in reactions in the other [21]. Peng and Simons noted that recombinant mosquito saliva allergens with biological activity were being developed and that these recombinant allergens will significantly improve diagnosis of mosquito allergies, eventually improving specific immunotherapy treatments for patients with systemic reactions to mosquito bites [20]. However, McCormack et al. mentioned that immunotherapy with whole body mosquito extracts is a viable treatment option that can play a role in patients with mosquito bite-induced anaphylaxis and that it might also result in severe side effects so one must determine the benefits versus the risks for each individual patient [21]. Reunala et al. stated that desensitization treatment is a theoretical possibility but prophylactically given cetirizine, an H1-blocking antihistamine, has been shown to be helpful for people suffering from mosquito bites [22]. Pharmacologically, cetirizine is a selective, second-generation histamine H1 receptor antagonist with a rapid onset, a long duration of activity, and a low potential for interaction with drugs metabolized by the hepatic cytochrome P450 system. Furthermore, cetirizine is generally more effective than other H1 receptor antagonists at inhibiting histamine-induced wheal and flare responses [23]. Curran et al. said that cetirizine is effective in the treatment of allergic cough and mosquito bites; however, its precise role in these indications has yet to be clearly established [23].

3. Medically Important Mosquitoes

Generally, mosquitoes can be found in all tropical countries. Although there are many mosquito species, only some species are considered medically important and only some species can be the vector of diseases. Mosquito-borne diseases, such as malaria and yellow fever, have been described in history for thousands of years. The transmission of pathogens by mosquitoes is dependent upon the relationship that exists between the pathogen, the invertebrate host (i.e., the mosquito vector), and the vertebrate host, each of which is influenced by environmental variations [24]. The frequency and extent of these diseases depends on a complex series of contributing factors. There have been several attempts to control mosquitoes. Many mosquito control agencies and health departments cooperate in being aware of the contributing factors in order to reduce the chances of disease.

A. *Aedes* Species

Aedes is a genus of mosquito that causes several tropical mosquito-borne diseases, including yellow fever, dengue virus infection, and filariasis. The mosquito, *Aedes aegypti*, is the primary worldwide arthropod vector for yellow fever and dengue viruses [25]. As it is also one of the most tractable mosquito species for laboratory studies, it has been—and remains—one of the most intensely-studied arthropod species [25]. Severson et al. reported that the research community is well-advanced in developing important molecular tools that may facilitate a whole genome sequencing effort [25]. They said that whole genome sequence information for *Aedes aegypti* would provide important insights into mosquito chromosome evolution and allow for the identification of genes and gene functions. Furthermore, these functions might be common to all mosquitoes or perhaps unique to individual species, possibly specific to host-seeking and blood-feeding behaviors as well as the innate immune response to pathogens encountered during blood feeding [25]. Black recently studied the genetic relationships among *Aedes aegypti* populations throughout the world and discussed how variation in vector competence is correlated with overall genetic differences among populations [26]. Black also described current research into how genetic and environmental factors jointly affect distribution of vector competence in natural populations [26]. Concerning the innate immune response of *Aedes aegypti*, Lowenberger said that an extremely effective response is part of the innate immunity exhibited by all insects and many invertebrates, and shows striking similarities with the innate immune response of vertebrates; however, not all insects utilize the same peptides in the same concentrations, which might reflect the pathogens to which they may have been exposed through evolutionary time [27]. Lowenberger noted that invasion of the hemocoel by bacteria in *Aedes aegypti* elicited the production of defensins and cecropins, peptides active only against gram-negative bacteria, and several other peptides [27]. They also noted the importance of those molecules involved in the response of *Aedes aegypti* to pathogens, and the potential role of these peptides against eukaryotic parasites that are ingested and transmitted by mosquitoes [27].

Concerning ecology of *Aedes aegypti*, this mosquito is considered a domestic mosquito. Rodhain noted that *Aedes aegypti* originated in Africa and expanded around the tropical world with a pantropical distribution in 1930 [28]. Rodhain noted that eggs of *Aedes aegypti* could survive unfavorable conditions, and larvae and pupae of *Aedes aegypti* bred in both natural and artificial containers [28]. Ordain said that artificial breeding sites are mostly water storage containers and discarded containers, where water is stored everywhere in Asia, including in large towns [28]. The control of water containers is therefore one of the most important components in the control of *Aedes aegypti*-borne diseases—especially dengue. Ordain noted that adult females of *Aedes aegypti* were mostly diurnal, indoor feeders, and adult densities were variable and could reach huge numbers [28]. Ordain mentioned that active dispersion of females was weak, with one female usually visiting one or two houses in its lifetime. The mean life duration of a female mosquito is about two to three weeks; thus, when infected with dengue virus and because of the duration of the extrinsic cycle of the virus, a female has a low probability of surviving long enough to transmit the disease [28].

The Asian tiger mosquito, or *Aides albopictus*, ranks second only to *Aedes aegypti* in importance to man as a vector of dengue and dengue hemorrhagic fever, which viruses place at risk a potential population of two billion people living in tropical and sub-tropical regions [29]. Gratz said that the mosquito *Aedes albopictus*, originally indigenous to Southeast Asia and islands of the Western Pacific and Indian Oceans, had spread during recent decades to Africa, the Mideast, Europe, and the Americas (both north and south) after extending its range eastwards across the Pacific islands during the early twentieth century [30]. Knudsen said that due to its predilection for breeding in a plethora of habitats within urban and suburban environs, as well as peri-rural areas, this mosquito is spreading rapidly where suitable breeding is available [29]. Knudsen noted that this mosquito exhibited strain differences ranging from cold-hardy to tropic-loving, yet despite limited flight range, it has spread beyond the Orient to China, the Pacific, the Indian Ocean islands, the Americas, parts of continental Africa and into southern Europe [29]. Kundsen said that this has been accomplished principally by means of transport of eggs in used tires via rapid air and sea transport [29]. Gratz noted that the majority of introductions were apparently due to transportation of dormant eggs in tires [30]. Knudsen also noted that egg-positive used tires, when shipped, and later rehydrated by rainfall, produced adult mosquitoes within a few days, rapidly infesting new areas [29]. Gratz reported that *Aedes albopictus* was a competent vector for at least 22 arboviruses [30]. Gratz also noted that there had been much concern that *Aedes albopictus* would lead to serious outbreaks of arbovirus diseases, notably dengue (all four serotypes) more commonly transmitted by *Aedes aegypti* [30]. Hudsen noted that *Aedes albopictus* was a potential vector of a number of arboviruses and could transmit them in a vertical or transvenereal manner in nature, thereby providing a means for their maintenance and transmission [29]. Gratz noted that results of many laboratory studies had shown that many arboviruses are readily transmitted by *Aedes albopictus* to laboratory animals and birds, and have frequently been isolated from wild-caught mosquitoes of this species, particularly in the Americas [30]. Gratz noted that *Aedes albopictus* probably served as a maintenance vector of dengue in rural areas of dengue-endemic countries of Southeast Asia and the Pacific islands, and he reported that *Aedes albopictus* also transmitted dog heartworm (*Dirofilaria immitis*) in Southeast Asia, southeastern USA, and both *Dirofilaria immitis* and *Dirofilaria repens* in Italy [30]. In the United States, Moore and Mitchell said that this mosquito had spread to 678 counties in 25 states since its discovery in Houston, Texas, in 1987 [31]. They said that although *Aedes albopictus*, a major biting pest throughout much of its range, was a competent laboratory vector of at least 22 arboviruses, including many viruses of public health importance, Cache Valley and eastern equine encephalomyelitis viruses were the only human pathogens isolated from U.S. populations of *Aedes albopictus* [31].

Aedes polynesiensis is a vector of human lymphatic filariasis [32]. Stolk et al. performed an interesting study to quantify the relationship between microfilaria density in human blood and the number of third stage (L3) larvae developing in mosquito vectors *Aedes polynesiensis* after blood-feeding [33]. According to this study, the average maximum number of L3 larvae that could develop into mosquitoes was estimated at 23 [33]. Lardeux and Cheffort said that among French Polynesian archipelagos where *Aedes polynesiensis* is the vector, the transmission potential for *Wuchereria bancrofti* and resulting disease manifestations of lymphatic filariasis in humans is correlated with ambient temperature due to the degree of southern latitude [34]. Burkot et al. mentioned that even with high mass drug administration (MDA) coverage, the efficiency of *Aedes polynesiensis* as a vector of *Wuchereria bancrofti* might limit the effectiveness of the elimination campaigns in some countries [35]. They also noted that in areas of limited MDA coverage, additional strategies, such as vector control (as an adjunct to MDA)—or alternative approaches, such as the use of diethylcarbamazine (DEC)-fortified salt—might be necessary to stop transmission [35].

B. Anopheles Species

Anopheles is a genus of mosquito that causes several tropical mosquito-borne diseases, especially malaria. Among the insects that serve as vectors for parasitic diseases, this genus is arguably the most important [36]. Of the approximately 400 species of *Anopheles*, about two dozen serve as vectors for malaria (*Plasmodium* spp.in humans); mosquitoes also serve as the vector for canine heartworm *(Dirofilaria immitis)* [36]. Several species of the *Anopheline* mosquito can be vectors of malaria. In 2004, Ool et al. performed a study to examine the species of *anopheline* mosquitoes in Myanmar and found that out of 36 species of *anophelines* distributed throughout the country, 10 species were found to be infected with the malarial parasite [37]. Gunasekaran et al. performed a similar study in the Koraput district of Orissa, India, which is highly malarious [38]. According to their study, a total of 62,086 *anophelines* belonging to 22 species and two varieties were collected, including 8 species of *anophelines* that are recognized malarial vectors in India [38]. In this study, a total of 24,154 mosquitoes were dissected and 18 mosquitoes belonging to four species, *Anopheles fluviatilis*, *Anopheles annularis*, *Anopheles culicifacies* and *Anopheles aconitus* were found with the gut/gland infection [38].

Norris said that human malaria was truly a disease of global proportions and was one of the most broadly distributed vector-borne infections and that *Anopheline* mosquitoes were the exclusive vectors of human malaria [39]. Norris noted that a handful of species predominated as the most notorious malarial vectors, but the species and forms involved in the transmission of human malaria worldwide were incredibly diverse [39]. Norris proposed that many of the *anophelines* that vector malaria existed as members of species complexes that often contain vector and nonvector species and that single *anopheline* species often exhibit significant heterogeneity across the species' range [39]. Norris said that this phenotypic and genotypic plasticity exacerbated the difficulties in identification of vector populations and implementation of effective surveillance and control strategies [39]. Norris mentioned that polytene chromosome investigations were among the first to provide researchers with tangible genetic markers that could be used to differentiate between what were recognized as species and chromosomal forms of *anopheline* mosquitoes [39]. Norris concluded that many new molecular markers have proven useful in a wide variety of applications including molecular taxonomy, evolutionary systematics, population genetics, genetic mapping, and investigation of defined phenotypes [39].

Concerning ecology of *anophilines*, there are several reports on this topic. Lien explained that of 25,656 specimens of *anopheline* mosquitoes collected by day from 1118 houses scattered over Taiwan Island, nearly 80% were *Anopheles minimus*, mostly from bedrooms [40]. Lien said that since the highly anthropophilic and endophilic *Anopheles minimus* was determined to be the chief vector of malaria in Taiwan, DDT was applied to the wall surfaces in houses for malarial control and eradication [40]. Herrel et al. performed an interesting study to understand how the population dynamics of adult *anopheline* mosquitoes could be related to malarial transmission in rural areas with intensive irrigation and a history of malarial epidemics [41]. They carried out a study in three villages located along an irrigation canal in South Punjab, Pakistan [41]. According to this study, *Anopheles subpictus* predominated (55.6%), followed by *Anopheles stephensi* (41.4%), *Anopheles culicifacies* (2.0%), *Anopheles pulcherrimus* (1.0%), and *Anopheles peditaeniatus* (0.1%) [41]. They reported that most mosquitoes (98.8%) were collected from indoor resting sites, whereas collections from potential resting sites outdoors accounted for only 1.2% of total *anopheline* densities, confirming the endophilic behavior of *anophelines* in Pakistan [41]. Herrel et al. concluded that, in South Punjab, irrigation-related sites supported the breeding of *anopheline* mosquitoes, including the vectors of malaria [41]. Das et al. studied the bioecology of *Anopheles philippinensis,* a vector of malaria on eight islands of the Andaman group [42]. It was found that *Anopheles philippinensis* preferred to rest and bite outdoors and that maximum biting was observed from 6 p.m. to 9 p.m. on both cattle and human bait [42]. Das et al. noted that the maximum breeding of *Anopheles philippinensis* was recorded in slow moving streams, followed by ponds with vegetation [42]. Depinay et al. recently performed a simulation model of African malarial vectors to examine different analyses and then conducted sensitivity analyses on temperature, moisture, predation and preliminary investigations of nutrient competition, and found many effects of the aforementioned factors [43]. In Southeast Asia, *Anopheles minimus* is mentioned as a major malarial vector, and it has become the main target of vector control in this area [44]. In rural areas, *Anopheles minimus* breeds along the banks of small, clear water streams [44]. Van Bortel et al. reported that there were *Anopheles minimus* mosquitoes whose immature stages develop in water tanks in the suburbs of Hanoi, northern Vietnam [44]. In 2003, Van Bortel et al. performed an interesting study on population genetic structure of the mosquito *Anopheles minimus* in Vietnam [44]. Van Bortel et al. noted that although significant genetic differentiation was observed between rural and urban *Anopheles minimus* populations, *Anopheles minimus* had not differentiated substantially by genetic drift [44]. Van Bortel et al. proposed that geographical distance is not the primary factor in differentiating *Anopheles minimus.* Populations having the typical breeding ecology and the estimated effective population size are consistent with moderate macrogeographical differentiation [44]. Van Bortel et al. concluded that the macrogeographical population structure indicates that genes might spread over large areas, whereas the presence of an urban *Anopheles minimus* population shows the ability of this species to adapt to anthropogenic environmental changes [44]. In addition to *Anopheles minimus*, *Anopheles dirus* is another important *anopheline* in Southeast Asia. This species is a problematic species with a high rate of drug resistance and it is widely distributed in Thailand and Myanmar [45]. This species is common in forest wood-extraction areas, irrigated plains areas near foothills, and coastal plains near foothill areas, as well as hilly areas [45].

C. *Culex* Species

The *Culex* mosquito, specifically the *Culex tarsalis*, has significance not only as a nuisance, but also as a potential carrier of many viruses, including West Nile virus, St. Louis encephalitis, and Western Equine encephalitis, the latter of which can be deadly to humans [46]. *Culex* mosquitoes are painful and persistent biters, which prefer to attack at dusk and after dark, and readily enter dwellings for blood meals [47]. A *Culex* mosquito can travel up to 25 miles from a breeding site, but generally stays close to its origin because winds in excess of six mph can inhibit its flight [46]. Domestic and wild birds are preferred prey over man, cows, and horses [47]. *Culex* are generally weak fliers and do not move far from home, although they have been known to fly up to two miles, and *Culex* mosquitoes usually live only a few weeks—about six weeks—during the warm summer months [46–47]. Gray and Bradley recently used flow-through respirometry on female *Culex* mosquitoes to observe individual ventilatory patterns and to measure metabolic rate at rest, during activity and after a blood-meal [48]. They found that blood feeding elicited a specific dynamic action lasting approximately 55 hours at the peak of which metabolic rate of the blood-fed females was twice that of the sugar-fed group [48]. They noted that an increase in metabolic rate presumably reflected the cost of blood digestion and egg production [48]. They also detected that the females were not active during digestion, so that although their metabolic rate was increased, the overall energy expenditure of the blood-fed group was not very different from that of the sugar-fed group [48].

The *Culex* mosquito lays her eggs in standing water, either foul or clear, and the habitats generally preferred are open, sunny areas, but shaded areas with vegetation are also used [46]. Similar to *Aedes aegypti*, the *Culex* mosquito is a container-breeding mosquito and the container may be as small as a flower vase or as large as an ornamental pond [46]. The egg-to-adult life cycle can be completed in seven to ten days, depending on the weather [46]. The water container is therefore an effective vector control for *Culex*.

Culex pipiens, or northern house mosquito, is the most common species of mosquito found in urban areas [46]. It appears to be primarily responsible for transmission of West Nile virus to humans and birds, as well as to other mammals [46]. Dohm et al. performed a study to investigate vertical transmission as a means of viral survival during interepizootics by intrathoracically inoculated *Culex pipiens* with West Nile virus and subsequently tested their F1 progeny for the presence of virus [49]. They found that female *Culex pipiens* that were vertically infected during the late summer season could serve as a source of West Nile virus to initiate an infection cycle the following spring [49]. Fouda et al. recently performed an interesting study to evaluate the influence of symbiotic bacteria associated with *Culex pipiens* on pre-oviposition and blood meal digestion period, reproductive potential, fecundity, and fertility [50]. According to this study, it seemed that the period of blood meal digestion preceded the pre-oviposition period of both bacterial-free females and bacterial-free females treated with one of the aforementioned bacteria [50]. Fouda et al. said that it is obviously clear that the presence of the two bacterial genera: *Bacillus* and *Staphylococcus* in the midgut of *Culex pipiens* is essential for normal and high fecundity, and it is evident that the symbionts (gut bacteria) are essential for the completion of embryonic development [50]. Dohm et al. also proposed that the effect of environmental temperature should to be considered when evaluating the vector competence of these mosquitoes and when modeling the risk of West Nile virus transmission in nature [51].

Culex quinquefasciatus is another important *Culex* mosquito. This mosquito is mentioned for its role in the transmission of *bancroftian filariasis*. *Culex quinquefasciatus* is usually indoor resting. Krishnamoorthy et al. said that the transmission success of the parasite might be reduced if the mosquitoes are highly loaded with parasites [52]. Dixit et al. recently studied *Culex quinquefasciatus* collected from three different habitats: human, cattle, and mixed dwellings of six localities of Raipur City in Madhya Pradesh state, India, for their sources of blood meal by precipitin test [53]. According to this study, of the 60 specimens from human dwellings, 52 were positive for human blood with an anthropophilic index of 90%; of the 25 specimens from cattlesheds, 15 were positive for human blood with an index of 60%; and of the 20 specimens from mixed dwellings, 12 showed human blood with an anthropophilic index of 63 % [53]. Dixit et al. concluded that the *Culex quinquefasciatus* of Raipur City is predominantly anthropophilic in nature irrespective of the nature of habitat of the mosquito vector [53]. In 2004, Samuel et al. performed another study to evaluate the host-feeding pattern of *Culex quinquefasciatus* and found that *Culex quinquefasciatus* is highly anthropophilic: human and cattle feeding accounted for 74.0% and 1.5% of the total bloodmeals tested, respectively [54]. They came to this conclusion from the high anthropophilic feeding rates of *Culex quinquefasciatus* collected from an endemic belt of Malayan filariasis, where epidemiological studies revealed the coexistence of *Bancroftian* and *Malayan filariasis* [54].

D. *Mansonia* Species

Mansonia species is an important group of mosquito that can carry many mosquito-borne diseases, especially lymphatic filariasis. The genus *Mansonia* is divided into two subgenera, *Mansonia* and *Mansonioides* [55]. The subgenus *Mansonioides* includes the important vectors of lymphatic filariasis caused by *Brugia malayi* in South and Southeast Asia [55]. Chiang noted that six species of this subgenus: *Mansonia bonneae*, *Mansonia dives*, *Mansonia uniformis*, *Mansonia annulifera*, *Mansonia annulata,* and *Mansonia indiana* are vectors of two types of brugian filariasis (periodic and subperiodic types) [55]. Concerning vector ecology, *Mansonia annulifera* was recorded to be an endophilic species, preferring to rest indoors; *Mansonia uniformis* is exophilic, having a predilection for outdoor resting habitats, such as bushes and shrubs; and *Mansonia indiana* did not show a clear preference to either of these biotopes [56]. Kumar et al. found that the unfed proportion of *Mansonia uniformis* in indoor resting collections was significantly higher during post-dusk compared to daytime hours, indicating that this exophilic species enters houses during dusk hours for feeding, and the full-fed proportion was higher during day hours compared to dusk/night hours [56]. Kumar et al. suggested that after having a blood-meal, this species rests indoors and leaves a house for outdoor resting sites during dusk hours on the subsequent night [56]. In 1984, Chiang et al. studied age groups within activity cycles, age composition, and survivorship in natural populations of *Mansonia* in Kampung Pantai, Bengkoka Peninsula of Sabah state, Malaysia [57]. According to this study, early activity of three to five parous *Mansonia bonneae* during the first hour after sunset was noted [57]. In addition, age composition of *Mansonia bonneae* in forest shade, indoor and outdoor of houses, and comparative buffalo versus human bait outdoor in Kampung Pantai showed all-around high parous rates ranging from 66.7% to 75.4% [57].

References

[1] McCartney, J. *Mosquitoes Taxonomy.* Available at http://www.personal.psu.edu/users/j/a/jam645/Taxonomy.htm.

[2] Maddison, D. R., W. P. Maddison, K.-S. Schulz, T. Wheeler, and J. Frumkin. 2001. *The Tree of Life Web Project.* Available at http://tolweb.org.

[3] Sutherland, D. J. *Mosquitoes in Your Life.* Available at http://www-rci.rutgers.edu/~insects/moslife.htm.

[4] Dieng, H., Mwandawiro, C., Boots, M., Morales, R., Satho, T., Tuno, N., Tsuda, Y. and Takagi, M. Leaf litter decay process and the growth performance of *Aedes albopictus* larvae (Diptera: Culicidae). *J. Vector. Ecol.* 27: 31–38 (2002).

[5] Chadee, D. D. Key premises.: A guide to *Aedes aegypti* (Diptera: Culicidae) surveillance and control. *Bull. Entomol. Res.* 94: 201-207 (2004).

[6] Lounibos, L. P., Suarez, S., Menendez, Z., Nishimura, N., Escher, R. L., O'Connell, S. M. and Rey, J. R. Does temperature affect the outcome of larval competition between *Aedes aegypti* and *Aedes albopictus*? *J. Vector. Ecol.* 27: 86–95 (2002).

[7] Wiwanitkit, V. and Suyaphan, A. The survey of malarial mosquito of Mae Suk subdistrict, Mae Jam, Chiangmai Province : A short report. *Lampang. Hosp. Bull.* 24 56–58 (2003).

[8] Shililu, J., Ghebremeskel, T., Seulu, F., Mengistu, S., Fekadu, H., Zerom, M., Asmelash, G. E., Sintasath, D., Mbogo, C., Githure, J., Brantly, E., Beier, J. C. and Novak, R. J. Seasonal abundance, vector behavior, and malaria parasite transmission in Eritrea. *J. Am. Mosq. Control. Assoc.* 20: 155–164 (2004).

[9] Edillo, F. E., Toure, Y. T., Lanzaro, G. C., Dolo, G. and Taylor, C. E. Survivorship and distribution of immature *Anopheles gambiae* s.l. (Diptera: Culicidae) in Banambani village. Mali. *J. Med. Entomol.* 41: 333–339 (2004).

[10] Shililu, J., Ghebremeskel, T., Mengistu, S., Fekadu, H., Zerom, M., Mbogo, C., Githure, J., Novak, R., Brantly, E. and, Beier, J. C. High seasonal variation in entomologic inoculation rates in Eritrea, a semi-arid region of unstable malaria in Africa. *Am. J. Trop. Med. Hyg.* 69: 607–613 (2003).

[11] Nirmala, X., Marinotti, O. and James, A. A. The accumulation of specific mRNAs following multiple blood meals in *Anopheles gambiae. Insect. Mol. Biol.* 14: 95–103 (2005).

[12] Dana, A. N., Hong, Y. S., Kern, M. K., Hillenmeyer, M. E., Harker, B. W., Lobo, N. F., Hogan, J. R., Romans, P. and Collins, F. H. Gene expression patterns associated with blood-feeding in the malaria mosquito *Anopheles gambiae. BMC. Genomics.* 6: 5 (2005).

[13] Smith, D. L., Dushoff, J. and McKenzie, F. E. The risk of a mosquito-borne infection in a heterogeneous environment. *PloS. Biol.* 2: e368 (2004).

[14] Mouchet, J. and Bellec, C. Recent achievements and perspectives in medical entomology and vector control. *Ann. Parasitol. Hum. Comp.* 65 (Suppl. 1): 107–111 (1990).

[15] Alekseev, A. N. Current problems in medical entomology. *Med. Parazitol. (Mosk).* 2: 7–10 (1999).

[16] Chow, C. Y. Medical entomology in Taiwan. *Gaoxiong. Yi. Xue. Ke. Xue. Za. Zhi.* 6: 322–324 (1990).

[17] Lehane, M. J. Vector insects and their control. *Ciba. Found. Symp.* 200: 8–16 (1996).

[18] Mulla, M. S. Mosquito control then, now, and in the future. *J. Am. Mosq. Control. Assoc.* 10: 574–584 (1994).

[19] Curtis, C. F. Approaches to vector control: New and trusted. 4. Appropriate technology for vector control: Impregnated bed nets, polystyrene beads and fly traps. *Trans. R. Soc. Trop. Med. Hyg.* 88: 144–146 (1994).

[20] Peng, Z., Simons, F. E. Mosquito allergy: Immune mechanisms and recombinant salivary allergens. *Int. Arch. Allergy. Immunol.* 133: 198–209 (2004).

[21] McCormack, D. R., Salata, K. F., Hershey, J. N., Carpenter, G. B. and Engler, R. J. Mosquito bite anaphylaxis: Immunotherapy with whole body extracts. *Ann. Allergy. Asthma. Immunol.* 74: 39–44 (1995).

[22] Reunala, T., Brummer-Korvenkontio, H. and Palosuo, T. Are we really allergic to mosquito bites? *Ann. Med.* 26: 301–306 (1994).

[23] Curran, M. P., Scott, L. J. and Perry, C. M. Cetirizine: A review of its use in allergic disorders. *Drugs.* 64: 523–561 (2004).

[24] Failloux, A. B., Vazeille-Falcoz, M., Mousson, L. and Rodhain, F. Genetic control of vectorial competence in *Aedes* mosquitoes. *Bull. Soc. Pathol. Exot.* 92: 266–273 (1999).

[25] Severson, D. W., Knudson, D. L., Soares, M. B. and Loftus, B. J. *Aedes aegypti* genomics. *Insect. Biochem. Mol. Biol.* 34: 715–721 (2004).

[26] Black, W. C. IV, Bennett, K. E., Gorrochotegui-Escalante, N., Barillas-Mury, C. V., Fernandez-Salas, I., de Lourdes Munoz, M., Farfan-Ale, J. A., Olson, K. E. and Beaty, B. J. Flavivirus susceptibility in *Aedes aegypti. Arch. Med. Res.* 33: 379–388 (2002).

[27] Lowenberger, C. Innate immune response of *Aedes aegypti. Insect. Biochem. Mol. Biol.* 31: 219–229 (2001).

[28] Rodhain, F. Ecology of *Aedes aegypti* in Africa and Asia. *Bull. Soc. Pathol. Exot.* 89: 103–106 (1996).

[29] Knudsen, A. B. Global distribution and continuing spread of *Aedes albopictus. Parassitologia.* 37: 91–97 (1995).

[30] Gratz, N. G. Critical review of the vector status of *Aedes albopictus. Med. Vet. Entomol.* 18: 215–227 (2004).

[31] Moore, C. G. and Mitchell, C. J. *Aedes albopictus* in the United States: Ten-year presence and public health implications. *Emerg. Infect. Dis.* 3: 329–334 (1997).

[32] *Aedes polyneniensis,* a vector of human lymphatic filariasis and *Aedes aegypti,* the vector of dengue viruses. *Bull. Soc. Pathol. Exot. 92:* 266–273 (1999).

[33] Stolk, W. A., Van Oortmarssen, G. J., Subramanian, S., Das, P. K., Borsboom, G. J., Habbema, J. D. and de Vlas, S. J. Assessing density dependence in the transmission of lymphatic filariasis: Uptake and development of *Wuchereria bancrofti* microfilariae in the vector mosquitoes. *Med. Vet. Entomol.* 18: 57–60 (2004).

[34] Lardeux, F. and Cheffort, J. Ambient temperature effects on the extrinsic incubation period of *Wuchereria bancrofti* in *Aedes polynesiensis:* Implications for filariasis transmission dynamics and distribution in French Polynesia. *Med. Vet. Entomol.* 15: 167–176 (2001).

[35] Burkot, T. R., Taleo, G., Toeaso, V. and Ichimori, K. Progress towards, and challenges for, the elimination of filariasis from Pacific-island communities. *Ann. Trop. Med. Parasitol.* 96 (Suppl. 2): S61–S69 (2002).

[36] *Anopheles* spp. Available at http://www.biosci.ohio-state.edu/~parasite/anopheles.html.

[37] Ool, T. T., Storch, V. and Becker, N. Review of the anopheline mosquitoes of Myanmar. *J. Vector. Ecol.* 29: 21–40 (2004).

[38] Gunasekaran, K., Sahu, S. S., Parida, S. K., Sadanandane, C., Jambulingam, P. and Das, P. K. Anopheline fauna of Koraput district, Orissa state, with particular reference to transmission of malaria. *Indian. J. Med. Res.* 89: 340–343 (1989).

[39] Norris, D. E. Genetic markers for study of the anopheline vectors of human malaria. *Int. J. Parasitol.* 32: 1607–1615 (2002).

[40] Lien, J. C. Anopheline mosquitoes and malaria parasites in Taiwan. *Gaoxiong. Yi. Xue. Ke. Xue. Za. Zhi.* 7: 207–223 (1991).

[41] Herrel, N., Amerasinghe, F. P., Ensink, J., Mukhtar, M., van der Hoek, W. and Konradsen, F. Adult anopheline ecology and malaria transmission in irrigated areas of South Punjab, Pakistan. *Med. Vet. Entomol.* 18: 141–152 (2004).

[42] Das, M. K., Nagpal, B. N., Srivastava, A. and Ansari, M. A. Bioecology of *An. philippinensis* in Andaman group of islands. *Vector. Borne. Dis.* 40: 43–48 (2003).

[43] Depinay, J. M., Mbogo, C. M., Killeen, G., Knols, B., Beier, J., Carlson, J., Dushoff, J., Billingsley, P., Mwambi, H., Githure, J., Toure, A. M. and McKenzie, F. E. A simulation model of African *Anopheles* ecology and population dynamics for the analysis of malaria transmission. *Malar. J.* 3: 29 (2004).

[44] Van Bortel, W., Trung, H. D., Roelants, P., Backeljau, T. and Coosemans, M. Population genetic structure of the malaria vector *Anopheles minimus* A in Vietnam. *Heredity.* 91: 487–493 (2003).

[45] Oo, T. T., Storch, V. and Becker, N. *Anopheles dirus* and its role in malaria transmission in Myanmar. *J. Vector. Ecol.* 28: 175–183 (2003).

[46] *Grand Forks Public Health Department. Mosquito.* Available at http://www.grandforksgov.com/publichealth/mosqua.htm.

[47] *Mosquito Homepage.* Available at www.montgomerycountymd.gov/content/dep/mosquito/facts.asp.

[48] Gray, E. M. and Bradley, T. J. Metabolic rate in female *Culex tarsalis* (Diptera: Culicidae): Age, size, activity, and feeding effects. *J. Med. Entomol.* 40: 903–911 (2003).

[49] Dohm, D. J., Sardelis, M. R. and Turell, M. J. Experimental vertical transmission of West Nile virus by *Culex pipiens* (Diptera: Culicidae). *J. Med. Entomol.* 39: 640–644 (2002).

[50] Fouda, M. A., Hassan, M. I., Al-Daly, A. G. and Hammad, K. M. Effect of midgut bacteria of *Culex pipiens* L. on digestion and reproduction. *J. Egypt. Soc. Parasitol.* 31: 767–780 (2001).

[51] Dohm, D. J., O'Guinn, M. L. and Turell, M. J. Effect of environmental temperature on the ability of *Culex pipiens* (Diptera: Culicidae) to transmit West Nile virus. *J. Med. Entomol.* 39: 221–225 (2002).

[52] Krishnamoorthy, K., Subramanian, S., Van Oortmarssen, G. J., Habbema, J. D. and Das, P. K. Vector survival and parasite infection: The effect of *Wuchereria bancrofti* on its vector *Culex quinquefasciatus. Parasitology.* 129 (Pt 1): 43–50 (2004).

[53] Dixit, V., Gupta, A. K., Kataria, O. M. and Prasad, G. B. Host preference of *Culex quinquefasciatus* in Raipur City of Chattisgarh state. *J. Commun. Dis.* 33: 17–22 (2001).

[54] Samuel, P. P., Arunachalam, N., Hiriyan, J., Thenmozhi, V., Gajanana, A. and Satyanarayana, K. Host-feeding pattern of *Culex quinquefasciatus* Say and *Mansonia annulifera* (Theobald) (Diptera: Culicidae), the major vectors of filariasis in a rural area of south India. *J. Med. Entomol.* 41: 442–446 (2004).

[55] Chiang, G. L. Update on the bionomics of *Mansonia* vectors of brugian filariasis. *Southeast. Asian. J. Trop. Med. Public. Health.* 24 (Suppl. 2): 69–75 (1993).

[56] Kumar, N. P., Sabesan, S. and Panicker, K. N. The resting and house-frequenting behavior of *Mansonia annulifera, Ma. Uniformis,* and *Ma. indiana,* the vectors of Malayan filariasis in Kerala State, India. *Southeast. Asian. J. Trop. Med. Public. Health.* 23: 324–327 (1992).

[57] Chiang, G. L., Cheong, W. H. and Samarawickrema, W. A. Filariasis in Bengkoka Peninsula, Sabah, Malaysia: Bionomics of *Mansonia* spp. *Southeast. Asian. J. Trop. Med. Public. Health.* 15: 294–302 (1984).

Chapter III

Control of Arbovirus Vector

Overview of Arthropod-borne Disease Control

To achieve success in the prevention and the control of the arthropod-borne illness, bringing up-to-date the data of those illnesses is necessary. Basic information is required before planning and launching any prevention strategy. New technology should be requested this purpose. Recently, Roberts and Rodriguez showed the value of the technology to in remote study of arthropod-borne illnesses [1]. They noted that many recent studies had also shown that it was necessary to completely define the environmental factors associated with the presence of spreading of vectors and illness, and to be capable of discerning these environmental factors with image data [1]. Singer and de Castro mentioned that required basic information for planning a successful prevention and control program for arthropod-borne illnesses should include data in interrelations among macro-political, economic and social politics, human migration, agricultural development, and transmission of the illness [2]. They also proposed the most useful of many spatial statistical methodologies connected with a geographical system of the information to describe the guidelines for human arrangement in the area, the ecological transformations induced by local professional practices, and the way in which these factors determine gradations of arthropod-borne infections that presented a risk [2].

Primary Prevention of Arboviral Infection

A. Vector Control

Vector control is a basic useful primary prevention method that can be applied to all arthropod-borne diseases. Because all arthropod-borne diseases are vector-borne diseases, the control of the vector is rational in prevention. Historically, Mulla said that the technology of control in the first half of the 20th century was relatively simple—reduction of the source that utilized fish of larvivorous types, hydrocarbon petroleums, and some synthetic, simple materials and botany. During the second half of the 20th century, nevertheless, several classes of synthetic organic chemical substances, improved formulations of the petroleum products, regulating synthetic pyrethroids, and microbic agents of control were developed and employed in the control of the arthropods and other illness-vectoring insects [3]. Mulla also noted that it was probable that those formulations of petroleum, insect growth regulators, and microbic agents of control would provide the main push against vectors, at least during the first quarter of the 21st century [3]. Various methods for the control of arthropod vectors are available at present.

B. Vaccination

Vaccination is available for some tropical arthropod-borne diseases, especially for Japanese encephalitis virus infection and yellow fever. The details of the vaccination in Japanese encephalitis and yellow fever are presented in the previous corresponding chapters. There are also several attempts to develop new vaccines for the other arthropod-borne diseases such as malaria, dengue infection and West Nile virus infection.

C. Zooprophylaxis

Zooprophylaxis is the diversion of insects to carry human illness to animals, and refers to control of vector-borne illnesses by attracting vectors to pets in which the pathogen cannot amplify out of the host. Zooprophylaxis is mentioned for the primary prevention of many contagious arthropod-borne illnesses. Zooprophylaxis has been proposed as a medium for the control of malaria since the beginning of the century to the present day [4]. Saul found that changing numbers of animals and accessibility had a small impact on the endemic and epidemic of the contagious arthropod-borne illness with the mortality of vector, but changing seek-associated behaviors and accessibility of humans had a greater effect. The most critical factor was the proximity of the animal to the arthropod. Saul concluded that zooprophylaxis might be ineffective with practical values of seek-associated mortality rates of the vector; nevertheless, the use of animals to attract the arthropods to the insecticide was predicted to be a promising strategy [5].

D. Control of Amplifying Host

The amplifying host plays an important role in the transmission of many arthropod-borne infectious diseases. Japanese encephalitis virus infection is a good example. An important amplifying host for Japanese encephalitis virus is the pig. The protection of pigs against arthropod-borne Japanese encephalitis by immunization with a live reduced vaccine is recommended. Sasaki et al. found that the vaccinated pigs developed circulating antibodies to Japanese encephalitis virus, and after challenges they did not develop viremia perceptible by inoculation of their serum in young mice, and they were also incapable of transmitting virus to arthropods that feed off the skin [6]. By contrast, unvaccinated pigs, when challenged by injection or by bites of arthropod, developed viremia and transmitted the virus to arthropods that were permitted to bite them [6]. With regard to the West Nile virus infection, the bird is mentioned as an important host that amplifies. The control of birds is necessary in this case. There are several attempts to vaccinate avians. Recently, Turell et al. evaluated a vaccine of DNA for the West Nile virus to determine if its use would be able to protect fish ravens (*Corvus ossifragus*) of the fatal West Nile virus infection [7]. In this study, the adult ravens captured were given 0.5 mg of this DNA vaccine orally or intramuscularly (IM); the ravens in the control group were exposed orally to a placebo [7]. Turell et al. found that although the oral administration of DNA vaccine as a single dose failed to remove an immune response or to protect the ravens from the West Nile virus infection, the IM administration of a single dose prevented death and associated viremia reduction [7]. In a severe outbreak, an important factor in the control of the amplifying host is destroying the suspected infected animals in the area of the outbreak.

Secondary Prevention of Arboviral Infection

Secondary prevention of arthropod-borne disease includes early diagnosis and prompt treatment of diseases, as previously mentioned. Kager reported that control of malaria is based on four principles: diagnosis and early processing; sustainable preventive and selective measures, including of the control of the vector; and discovery, contention and prevention of epidemics and building local capacity [8]. With regard to the infection of dengue fever virus, Rodriguez-Tann and Weir said that once a person is infected, the key to survival is early diagnosis and appropriate processing for severe cases with complications of life-threatening dengue fever, dengue hemorrhagic fever and dengue shock syndrome [9]. Guzman and Kouri said that appropriate rapid, early and accessible useful diagnosis for epidemiological caution and clinical diagnosis were still needed [10].

Advents in Control of Arbovirus Vector

With advents in genetic medicine, there are many new advents in control of arbovirus vectors. When an arbovirus enters an arthropod in an infected blood meal, several mechanisms may interact to affect its life cycle and ultimate transmissibility [11]. Intrinsic absolute failure in the establishment of infection must be contrasted with infection that is successfully established but is variably modulated in its viral yield throughout the vector's life span [11]. Murphy said that human intervention that affects modulating mechanisms may become a basis for disease control [11]. It is now accepted that genetic manipulation of arbovirus vector can profoundly and permanently reduce their competence to transmit the viruses to human hosts. For example, the dengue-resistant mosquito is being successfully manipulated at present [12]. Modern molecular approaches will undoubtedly provide considerable information about gene regulation and expression in vectors and consequently a much better understanding of the biology and molecular biology of vectors [13]. Such knowledge is essential for developing effective control strategies for vector-borne diseases [13].

References

[1] Roberts DR, Rodriguez MH. The environment, remote sensing, and malaria control. *Ann. N. Y. Acad. Sci.* 740, 396-402 (1994)

[2] Singer BH, de Castro MC. Agricultural colonization and malaria on the Amazon frontier. *Ann. N. Y. Acad. Sci.* 954,184-222 (2001)

[3] Mulla MS. Arthropod control then, now, and in the future. *J. Am. Mosq. Control. Assoc.* 10:574-84 (1994)

[4] Bettini S, Romi R. Zooprophylaxis: old and new problems. *Parassitologia.* 40, 423-30 (1998)

[5] Saul A. Zooprophylaxis or zoopotentiation: the outcome of introducing animals on vector transmission is highly dependent on the arthropod mortality while searching. *Malar. J.* 2, 32 (2003)

[6] Sasaki O, Karoji Y, Kuroda A, Karaki T, Takenokuma K, Maeda O. Protection of pigs against arthropod-borne Japanese encephalitis virus by immunization with a live attenuated vaccine. *Antiviral. Res.* 2, 355-60 (1982)

[7] Turell MJ, Bunning M, Ludwig GV, Ortman B, Chang J, Speaker T, Spielman A, McLean R, Komar N, Gates R, McNamara T, Creekmore T, Farley L, Mitchell CJ. DNA vaccine for West Nile virus infection in fish crows (Corvus ossifragus). *Emerg. Infect. Dis.* 9, 1077-81 (2003)

[8] Kager PA. Malaria control: constraints and opportunities. *Trop. Med. Int. Health.* 7, 1042-6 (2002)

[9] Rodriguez-Tan RS, Weir MR. Dengue: a review. *Tex. Med.* 94, 53-9 (1998)

[10] Guzman MG, Kouri G. Dengue diagnosis, advances and challenges. *Int. J. Infect. Dis.* 8, 69-80 (2004)

[11] Murphy FA. Cellular resistance to arbovirus infection. *Ann. N. Y. Acad. Sci.* 266, 197-203 (1975)

[12] Olson KE, Adelman ZN, Travanty EA, Sanchez-Vargas I, Beaty BJ, Blair CD. Developing arbovirus resistance in mosquitoes. *Insect. Biochem. Mol. Biol.* 32, 1333-43 (2002)

[13] Carlson J, Olson K, Higgs S, Beaty B. Molecular genetic manipulation of mosquito vectors. *Annu. Rev. Entomol.* 40:359-88 (1995)

Chapter IV

Dengue Infection

Introduction to Dengue Infection

Dengue infection is a mosquito-borne arboviral infection. Dengue fever viral infection includes a variable spectrum of illness that ranges from a simple fever to severe dengue hemorrhagic fever (HDF), a fatal disease [1]. Mairuhu et al. said that dengue fever came to be more recognized as one of the more significant contagious illnesses of the world due to increased incidence and spreading geographical distribution of dengue fever in the last 50 years [1]. Nogueira said that dengue fever was one of the very frequent predominant acute contagious illnesses and might be extremely fatal if associated with complications [2]. Halstead said that the antibodies played important roles in protection and virulence of infections of dengue fever; therefore, studies to determine which cells are infected in human dengue fever, along with comprehension of early antibody-accessible steps of the infection, should concentrate on the cellular level [3]. Nogueira also noted that control of the vector was still the most effective measure [2]. Although there been many efforts during the last six decades to produce a vaccine to fight this infection, few have been capable of meeting the challenges placed by the exceptional interaction between this virus and its human host [4]. Owing to present-day globalization, dengue fever has emerged as an arising contagious problem not only in tropical but also in nontropical countries. Wilson recently said that travelers could also be seen as messengers that transport pathogens and microbial genetic matter to other regions where investigators could carry out detailed analyses that could help map the location and movement of strains, genotypes and resistance patterns [5]. Knowledge of dengue infection is, therefore, an interesting theme for general practitioners throughout the world.

Worldwide Epidemiology of Dengue Infection

Dengue viral infection is one of the most important mosquito-borne illnesses throughout the world. Currently, dengue fever is reported in more than 100 countries. Malavige noted that 100 million cases of dengue fever and a half million cases of DHF occur yearly worldwide [6]. More than ninety percent of infected subjects are children less than 15 years old [6]. This illness is classified as a tropical illness with extremely endemic area in Southeast Asia. Nevertheless, the spread of the illness to other regions is reported. Globalization is an important factor as indicated previously. In 2003, Guzman and Kouri reported that epidemiological situation in Latin America seemed similar to that of Southeast Asia [7]. In 2002, Guzman and Kouri also reported a comparison in incident and fatality rates of dengue infection in three regions: Southeast Asia, Western Pacific, and Americas. According to this study, similar patterns in three regions were able to be observed [8]. Finally, Menard noted that this illness had scattered through the tropical region in the past forty years, beyond its original site in Southeast Asia [9]. Menard also noted that it sometimes has appeared in a severe form as DHF, which requires specialized medical care in some geographical areas [9]. A summary of some recent reports on dengue epidemiology in several regions of the world is hereby presented.

A. Asia

Asia is an endemic area of dengue infection. As previously described, the peak incidence is reported in Southeast Asian countries. In 2001, Corwin et al. investigated an outbreak of dengue infection in Palembang, southern Sumatra, Indonesia [10]. According to this study, an apparent tendency in the spread of the epidemic was observed, evolving from a cyclic phenomenon from five years to an often indistinguishable, annual occurrence from one year to the next [10]. They reported that proportional distribution of clinical epidemic cases in dengue fever, DHF and the dengue shock syndrome (DSS) were 24%, 66%, and 10%, respectively [10]. They also found that the population aged 10–19 years justified the largest proportion (35%) of hospitalized cases of DHF, followed by children aged 5–9 years (25%) and children aged 4 years (16%) [10]. Tuntaprasart et al. reported another interesting report of outbreak of dengue fever that occurred in Muang District, Ratchaburi Province, Thailand in 2001 [11]. According to this outbreak, about 800 cases of infection were reported, and among them, 49.5% were diagnosed clinically as DHF [11]. In this study, a seroepidemiological inspection was carried out among 283 primary students, to control spreading of dengue fever [11]. According to this study, an increase in the rate of seroconversion was observed in the period from September to December 2000, while the peak of outbreak occurred in the dry season, February 2001 [11]. Tuntaprasart et al. concluded that serosurveys among students appeared be early warning system, and could be profitable in early actions for control of dengue fever, breaking chain of spreading before an imminent epidemic [11]. Pinheiro said that DHF had continued to show a higher incidence in Southeast Asia in the 1990s, especially in Viet Nam and Thailand, which accounted for more than two thirds of cases of DHF reported in Asia [12]. With regard to the other parts of Asia, the infection of dengue can be also seen. In Southern Asia, there are many reports on the epidemiology of dengue fever from India. In 2004, Shah et al. reported that endemicity of dengue fever was on the rise in Mumbai with an increased incidence among children [13]. Moreover, a case of dengue fever was reported for the first time in a rural area of Kurnool District, Andhra Pradesh, India in 2004 [14]. Entomological and serological investigations were carried out to determine the frequency of vectors of dengue fever and dengue fever virus [14]. Arunachalam et al. found that larval indices for *Aedes aegypti* were manifested in the following way: house index 28–40%, container index 13–37%, and Breteau index 32–60 [14]. For nontropical Asia, the infection of dengue was also reported in recent years. In eastern Asia, China—a temperate Asian country—also faces infection of dengue as a new emerging contagious illness in the present [15]. Recently, Luo et al. noted that a sum of 9,747 cases of dengue fever was reported, with three deaths in the province of Guangdong, 1990–2000 [16]. They noted that the epidemic of dengue fever in Guangdong was closely related to the neighboring countries, indicating the possibility of importing the virus from those countries, and that epidemics generally begin with imported infected cases [16].

B. North America

In the past, North America was considered as a dengue fever-free region. Nevertheless, dengue infection came to be a significant emerging imported infection in the past few years. Within the last decade, an unheard-of occurrence of an epidemic of dengue fever in the American hemisphere was witnessed. DeHart said that vectors of yellow fever, malaria, and dengue fever could be identified in airplanes, and they should be considered an important matter of travel medicine in airplanes [17]. Pinheiro said that an epidemic of DHF occurred in the Americas in 1981, almost 30 years after their appearance in Asia, and their incidence showed a marked upward trend [12]. Pinheiro noted that a main cause of the emergence of DHF in the Americas was the failure of the hemispherical campaign to eradicate *Aedes aegypti.*

C. Latin America and South America

There are many recent reports on the dengue infection epidemiology of Latin America and South America. Reiskind et al. recently carried out a serological, environmental and epidemiological inspection to determine the risk factors in Peru [18]. According to this study, in general terms, the frequency of antibody was about 29%, and more than doubled from the youngest to the oldest age groups, but did not differ according to gender [18]. Curiously, the length of residence in Santa Clara was negatively associated with dengue fever virus antibodies [18]. They found that those who obtained water from a river source rather than a local well also had a significantly higher antibody rate and none of the environmental variables measured at each household related to the antibody distribution pattern [18]. Reiskind et al. suggested that a recent outbreak of dengue fever virus did not occur in the village, and that a majority of infections among residents of this rural village were acquired by visiting Iquitos city [18]. Vaughn carried out another interesting retrospective study on outbreaks of dengue fever in Cuba [19]. Vaughn found that all patients with symptomatic dengue fever, including of 205 cases of DHF and 12 deaths, were adults born before the dengue virus type 1 epidemic, and almost all (98%) experienced secondary infections of dengue virus [19]. In 1981, Cuba reported the first outbreak of DHF in Latin America, during which a total of 344,203 cases of dengue fever were identified, including 10,312 severe cases and 158 deaths [12]. DHF in the Cuban epidemic was associated with dengue fever-2 virus and occurred four years after dengue fever-1 had been introduced into the area [12]. Pinheiro said that growth and rapid urbanization of populations in Latin America and the Caribbean, and increased travel of persons who facilitate dengue fever virus dissemination, were important factors contributing to the emergence of the infection in these countries [12].

D. Europe

Similar to North America, the infection of dengue fever virus has been imported in Europe for the past few years. Haas et al. noted that some arising contagious illnesses including dengue infection had recently become endemic in Germany [20]. They also noted that outbreaks of dengue fever in new endemic areas could be due to infections detected in travelers who return from the original endemic areas [20]. Badiaga et al. recently carried out an interesting retrospective study on imported dengue fever virus infection in France [21]. They found that infection was observed more in feverish travelers who returned from tropical areas, especially those who returned from the Caribbean islands and Southeast Asia, but it was rarely diagnosed in travelers who returned from Africa [21]. In a retrospective study of 44 cases of imported infection of dengue fever diagnosed in France, Badiaga et al. found that the epidemiology, clinical characteristics and diagnoses of these cases were similar to those reported in other prior studies published [21]. Gascon et al. carried out another study in 57 Spanish travelers with the infection of imported dengue fever [22]. In this report, all patients had traveled to endemic areas (Central America, 28 cases; Indian subcontinent, 15; Southeast Asia, 10; South America, 2; Western Africa, 1; and Pacific, 1) [22]. The most important clinical characteristics were described as follows: fever and asthenia (100%), headache (98%), myalgia (84%), arthralgia (72%), rash (61%) and retroocular pain (65%) [22]. Gascon et al. noted that dengue fever should be included in the differential diagnosis of dengue fever in patients who return from trips to tropical areas [22].

E. Africa

The infection of dengue fever virus is also documented in Africa. In the past, the dengue fever 1 and 2 viruses were mentioned for most African cases [24]. In 1977, the neutralization tests carried out in 1,816 humans living in different geographical locations in Nigeria by Fagbami et al. showed that 45% of Nigerians were immunized to dengue fever-2 virus [24]. The first known outbreak of dengue fever-3 virus in Africa was documented by the isolation of virus during an epidemic of dengue fever-like illness in Pemba, Mozambique, in late 1984 and early 1985 [24]. In 1995, Rodier et al. said that sanitary priorities in the quickly-growing city of Djibouti in eastern Africa had been altered for many contagious illnesses, including malaria, AIDS, tuberculosis, dengue fever and cholera, which were under control until the early 1980s [25]. They said that poverty seemed to be a greater cause for the exit and the reappearance of these contagious illnesses [25].

F. Australia

The infection of dengue fever virus is considered an important emerging illness in Australia [26]. Russell and Dwyer said that mosquito-borne arboviruses were an important sanitary matter in Australia [27]. They noted that virus of dengue fever was detected in some areas of Australia [27]. In Queensland, there have been many reports on the epidemiology of dengue fever [28]. Malcolm et al. noted that general practitioners should immediately report all clinically suspected cases of dengue fever in travelers recently arriving in north Queensland [28]. In 2002, Hills et al. reported a recent outbreak of dengue infection in two suburbs in Townsville, north Queensland [29]. The serogroup of dengue fever-2 were the causative virus, and nine cases of dengue fever were documented [29].

Vector and Transmission

The infection of dengue fever is a viral, tropical and important illness. Dengue fever is an illness of arbovirus (group B), transmitted by *Aedes aegypti*, a mosquito that feeds inside [30]. With regard to the illnesses of arbovirus, most of the arboviruses that affects humans are included in the families *Togaviridae*, *Flaviviridae*, *Bunyaviridae*, *Reoviridae* and *Rhabdoviridae* [31]. Many infections of arbovirus are symptomless [31]. The clinical manifestation ranges from mild feverish illness, with or without skin rash and arthralgia, to more fatal and severe encephalitis or hemorrhagic complications. The virus of dengue fever is classified in the family *Flaviviridae*. In additional to virus of dengue fever, yellow fever virus and Japanese encephalitis (JE) virus are the other two medically-important arboviruses [31]. With respect to virus of dengue fever, four main serogroups, dengue fever-1, -2, -3 and -4 are documented. As previously mentioned, the infection of dengue fever virus is a mosquito-borne infection. *Aedes aegypti* is the vector of dengue fever. About two thirds of the world population live in areas infested with vectors of dengue fever, mainly *Aedes aegypti* [12]. All four dengue viruses are circulating, sometimes simultaneously, in most of these areas [12]. Degallier et al. said that bioecological parameters that were of special importance in the epidemiology of the infection include three levels: nature of *Aedes aegypti*-human contacts, sensitivity of pathogenic mosquito and multiplication of pathogen, and transmission [32] (Table 1).

Table 1. Bioecological parameters that are of special importance in the epidemiology of dengue infection [32]

Parameters	Factors
1. vector-human contact	trophic preferences, density variations, daily survival rate, egg diapause, human influences
2. susceptibility and multiplication	temperature, genetical nature of viral and mosquito strains
3. transmission	temperature, genetic

Wiwanitkit V, 2005.

Besides simple transmission by vector, other ways of simple transmission for dengue infection are also documented. Some pregnant women can also be susceptible to dengue fever and if they experience the infection of dengue fever virus, the vertical transmission of the virus their babies can be expected. The intrapartum infection is an interesting tropical intrapartum infection. There are some prior reports on this kind of intrapartum infection. The vertical transmission due to the infection of dengue fever during pregnancy was first reported by Thaithumyanon et al. in 1994 [33]. The intrapartum infection can bring several complications, mainly due disorders of coagulation. With regard to the clinical presentation of the affected pregnant subjects, similar presentation to general population can be seen [34]. It can be noted that the intrapartum and postnatal disorders of coagulation cascades can be corrected by the replacement therapy. Of interest, intrapartum complications were dependant to postpartum complications. Besides, it seems that complications did not relate to method of the delivery. Truly, confirmation for intrapartum dengue infection is generally after due to the long turnaround time of the serological test. Firstly, a bacterial infection was suspected initially in most cases. Nevertheless, the presumed diagnosis is generally due to combined presentation of fever and thrombocytopenia. Truly, in areas where infection of dengue fever virus is endemic, the diagnosis of dengue fever should be considered in neonates with signs of the bacterial infection [35-36]. When fever is suspected in a pregnant woman, the laboratory investigation and prolonged observation of newborn are advised [35 – 36]. Due to possible long time expected for results of laboratory investigation, beginning replacement therapy in clinically suspected cases is recommended. After the final diagnosis, mother and baby should be closely followed up.

Genetic and Molecular Biology of Dengue Infection

The transmission of pathogens by arthropods is a key in the relations that exist among pathogen, invertebrate host or vector and vertebrate host, each one that is influenced by environmental variations [37]. Genetic is one of important intrinsic factors and mechanisms that control the ability of vectors to transmit pathogens [37]. Polymorphism in expression of sensitivity to oral infection has been shown to occur among geographical samples of mosquitoes [37]. Failloux et al. said that it had been tested for specific variations of competence of vector and it could be shown that they were controlled by one or more genes and aforesaid in variable proportions inside a population of the mosquito [37]. They also noted that recent advances in the molecular biology had facilitated accessibility of nucleic acid data [37]. At present, little is known about role of vector in diffusion of virus of dengue fever [38]. There are some recent reports that utilized allozyme polymorphism investigations for genetic variations of vector of dengue fever from many countries. For example, Failloux et al. studied genetic pattern of vector of dengue fever in French Polynesia [38]. According to this study, low level of genetic changed among populations of mosquito in different islands [38]. Failloux et al. concluded that occurrence of dengue hemorrhagic fever in French Polynesia during the last few years was probable due to the dispersal of the dengue virus via viremic people rather than via infected vectors [38]. Gorrochotegui-Escalante et al. carried out another interesting study in Mexico [39]. In this study, a genetic analysis was carried out among 10 collections of *Aedes aegypti* of seven cities on the coast of northeast Mexico [39]. Four collections were gathered from Monterrey to examine local patterns of gene flow [39]. Sixty random samples of amplified polymorphic DNA (RAPD) loci were amplified by polymerase chain reaction and single-strand conformation polymorphism analysis of variation in a 387-basepair region of the NADH dehydrogenase subunit 4 from the mitochondrial DNA (mtDNA) [39]. According to this study, regression analysis of geographic distances and pairwise FST estimated from RAPD markers indicated isolation by distance and that liberated gene flow occurred among collections within 90–250 km [39]. Finally, Tran et al. carried out a study on sensitivity of vector of dengue fever-2 virus and its genetic differentiation in Vietnam [40]. They studied tangibility in the competence of *Aedes aegypti* as a vector for dengue fever-2 virus and genetic differentiation in this mosquito species [40]. In this study, 20 samples of the mosquito collected in 1998 in Ho Chi Minh City were subject to oral infection, and analysis of isoenzyme polymorphism by starch gel electrophoresis was performed [40]. Tran et al. found that those populations of *Aedes aegypti* in the center of the city were genetically differentiated, and their rates of infection differed from those populations in exterior neighborhood zones [40].

Besides genetic pattern of vector, the effect of genetic polymorphism in humans is of interest. Among the several advanced hypotheses to explain the pathogenesis of severe dengue fever, the model of immunopathogenesis is the majority that mention a probable important role played by cytokine cascades [41]. In 2004, Fernandez-Mestre et al. described polymorphism of tumor necrosis factor (TNF)-alpha, interferon-gamma, interleukin (IL)-6, and transforming growth factor-beta1 in patients with dengue fever virus infections and analyzed the relation with clinical manifestations of the illness [41]. In conclusion, they reported a possible association among high levels of circulating TNF to vascular permeability and hemorrhage in the patients with DHF [41]. There was another interesting study in Vietnam in 2002 [42]. In that study of the case-control in 400 patients with DHF and 300 matched controls, Left et al. valued five polymorphic non-HLA host genetic factors that might influence sensitivity to DHF [42]. They found that the less frequent *t* allele of a variant at position 352 of the vitamin D receptor (VDR) gene was related to resistance to severe fever [42]. They also discerned that homozygotes for arginine variant in position 131 of the gene of Fc gamma RIIA had less capacity to opsonize IgG2 antibodies and might also protect from DHF [42]. Nevertheless, they did not find associations with polymorphisms in the mannose binding lectin, interleukin-4 (IL-4), and IL-1 receiver antagonist genes [42].

Pathophysiology and Clinical Manifestation

A. Pathophysiology of Dengue Infection

Dengue fever is a viral illness with clinical characteristics that vary in intensity according to host and viral characteristics [43]. Truly, the infection of dengue fever virus is generally a nonspecific feverish illness that is resolved with the supporting therapy with a clinical spectrum from asymptomatic infection to hemorrhage and sudden death [44]. The pathophysiology of severe forms of dengue fever can be related to sequential infection with different serogroups, variations in the virulence of virus, interaction of virus with environmental and host factors or a combination of these factors [44]. Courageot et al. noted that result of dengue virus infection depends on viral and host factors and cells of host were thought to respond to viral infection by initiation of death of the cell or apopsis [45]. Courageot et al. said that there was evidence that dengue fever virus could cause cell of host to experience apoptosis in a cell-dependent way then virally induced apoptosis contributed directly to the cytopathogenic effects of dengue virus in cultured cells then the induction of apoptosis involves the activation of intracellular signaling systems [45]. Courageot et al. said that cellular factors that regulate cell death, such as members of the Bcl-2 family, could modulate the outcome of dengue virus infection in cultured cells, and apoptosis inhibitors delayed dengue virus-induced apoptosis, thereby providing a suitable environment for the virus [45]. They concluded that death of the cell was also modulated by the virulence of the infecting strains during dengue virus infection [45].

In a severe form of dengue fever, DHF, the immune response of host is important factor in course of illness [46]. These responses are immune complex formation, activation of complement, increase histamine liberation and massive liberation of many cytokines into the circulation, carrying shock, vasculopathy, thrombopathy and diffused intravascular coagulation (DIC) [46]. Nevertheless, fundamental mechanisms of severe bleeding in DHF are not completely understood. Recently, Falconar proposed that dengue virus nonstructural-1 protein (NS1) generated antibodies to common epitopes on human blood clotting and integrin/adhesin proteins on thrombocytes [47]. Falconar found that anti-NS1 polyclonal antisera reacted with the NS1 proteins of the dengue virus, but only weakly reacted with the NS1 proteins of the other flaviviruses [47]. Besides, various antibodies of monoclonal anti-NS1 produced hemorrhage in mice, cross-reacted with human fibrinogen, thrombocytes and endothelial cells, with known epitopes or active places in human coagulation factors and integrin/adhesin proteins present in these cells [47]. In 1995, Wang et al. reported the first evidence of dengue fever-2 tied to human platelets only in the presence of virus-specific antibody, maintaining a role for immune-mediated clearance of platelets in the pathogenesis of thrombocytopenia in DHF [48]. It is mentioned that responses of antibody engendered by mice to protein of dengue fever NS1 were influenced by the MHC class II (I-A) haplotype but each antiserum cross-reacted with human fibrinogen, thrombocytes and endothelial cells [47]. In a recent study, dengue fever NS1 protein presents closed phylogenetic correlation to CD61 that fibrinogen and other two integrin/adhesin proteins of platelet (CD41 and CD49B) [49]. Truly, Chang et al. reported that dengue fever NS1 immobilized in the coverslips had as a result more cell adhesion than did the control proteins, and indicated that integrin-relating peptides' structural mimicry existed within the NS1 antigen [50]. Moreover, Wiwanitkit carried out recently an in silico study for the homologue between the sequence of amino acid of NS1 and human integrin [51]. Wiwanitkit proposed that integrin/adhesin proteins of platelet, especially CD61, might play an important role to cause hemorrhagic complication in the infection of dengue fever virus [51]. Therefore, facts on platelet CD61 should be focused in the additional study in its role in the pathogenesis of DHF [51]. With regard to the most severe form of dengue fever, DSS, complicated pathophysiology is mentioned. The lei et al. noted that the hypothesis of the antibody-dependent increase, of virulence of virus, and of the gamma of IFN/immunopathogenesis halfway through of TNFalpha was insufficient to explain the clinical manifestations of DHF/DSS just as thrombocytopenia and hemoconcentration [52]. Lei et al. proposed a new hypothesis for the immunopathogenesis for dengue fever virus infection that aberrant immune answers did not only damage the immune response to empty virus, but also had a result as overproduction of cytokines that affected monocytes, cells of endothelium, and hepatocytes [52]. They proposed that platelets were destroyed by crossreactive anti- platelet autoantibodies [52]. They also said that vasculopathy and coagulopathy induced by virus should be implied in the patogenesis of hemorrhage, and the unbalances between activation of coagulation and fibrinolysis increased probability of severe hemorrhage in the DHF/DSS [52]. They noted that hemostasis was maintained unless the dysregulation of coagulation and fibrinolysis persist and the overproduced IL-6 might played a crucial role in the enhanced production of anti-platelet or anti-endothelial cell autoantibodies, elevated levels of tPA, as well as a deficiency in coagulation [52]. Besides, capillary shrinkage was caused by the dengue fever virus or by antibodies responding to antigens [52]. Lei et al. concluded that immunopathogenesis of DHF/DSS would be able to justify specific characteristics of epidemiological, pathological, and clinical observations in this viral infection [52]. Rodriguez-Ortega proposed another interesting hypothesis for the development of severe infection of dengue fever virus including DSS [53]. Rodriguez-Ortega noted that nitric oxide (NO), a polyvalent molecule that implies in processes of cytotoxic as well as cytoprotective, was extremely regulated by the cell because a modification in any production associated with a variety of pathologies including hemorrhagic shock in the infection of dengue fever virus [53].

B. Clinical Manifestation of Dengue Infection

Dengue infection is a common tropical disease with mosquito vector. Concerning the infection, the classical description is an incubation period of five to eight days followed by the onset of a fever, violent headache, chills, with a rash developing after three to four days. Generally, most of the infections of dengue fever virus are classified as dengue fever, generally presented with fever with constitutional symptoms and positive tourniquet test [7-8, 54]. The high fever generally lasts four to seven days, and the majority of people have a complete recovery without complications [7-8, 54] (Table 2). Nevertheless, it can show several atypical forms without fever or clinically significant symptoms [7-8, 54]. According to a recent study in Thailand, the fever was the most common presentation of the patients (100%) [55]. These conclusions are similar to recent report of an epidemic in Delhi [56]. Of interest, the respiratory and gastrointestinal symptoms such as vomiting and coughs presented in a few Thai studied population [55]. Truly, fever is one of hallmarks for diagnosis of the infection of dengue fever virus [7-8, 54]. Unfortunately, several tropical illnesses present with fever, therefore, this complaint is not specific and useless in clinical practice. With regard to characteristics of patients of different degree of severity (Table 3): dengue fever, DHF and DSS in a recent study of Wiwanitkit, some notable conclusions should be discussed. First, the mean age of patients in each category progressively increased as the category of illness moved from less to more severe disease, nevertheless, this tendency is not statistically significant [55]. Second, the hematocrit progressively increases due to increasing hemoconcentration of the illness. Nevertheless, there is no statistically significant difference between DHF and DSS [55]. Last, platelet count is lower for DHF and DSS [55].

Concerning the fever, high-grade fever (average >38°C) is a hallmark of the infection [7-8, 57]. A history of high fever that is not relieved by ingestion of self-prescribed acetaminophen could be a useful point for the general practitioner in the tropical countries that are faced with those patients in the endemic season. Concerning the correlation between body temperature and total white blood cell count and differential white blood cell count, non-significant correlation could be detected. Therefore, the fever and the lymphocytosis in the patients with dengue fever is only a copresentation. Although the fever is believed to due to the cytokine excreted from the lymphocyte the lymphocyte count is not relating to the body temperature level. As already mentioned, the explanation might be due to the fact that the patients usually got the antipyretic drug before visiting the physician, which can be the modifying factor for the body temperature. The pattern of dengue fever also varies on the date of infection as well (Table 2).

With regard to the hematological manifestation of dengue infection, there are various important hematological findings. Thrombocytopenia and hypofibrinogenemia are two common defects of the hemostasis [58]. Increased intravascular coagulation seems to be a responsible factor, although not an outstanding one [58].

Table 2. Phase of dengue infection

Phase	Day	Brief description
Febrile phase	1–2	High fever (usually more than 38°C), erythrema, myalgia, nausea, vomiting, sore throat, petichiae, positive tourniquet test, hepatomegaly, local lymphadenopathy (elbow fossa)
Toxic phase	3–5	Abruptly decreased fever, weak pulse, restlessness, blood pressure dropping, abdominal pain, positive tourniquet test, pending shock*
Convalescent phase	6–7	Recovery from illness, decreased hepatomegaly, positive tourniquet test

Wiwnitkit V, 2005.

* It should be noted that DSS can be seen only in the case with secondary heterotypic infection.

Table 3. Summary of important clues for discrimination for three degrees of severity of dengue infection

Grade	Blood pressure	Some clinical notes
Grade I	Normal	Only positive tourniquet test
Grade II	Normal	Some bleeding presentations
Grade III	Decrease	Severe, can detect blood pressure
Grade IV	Decrease	Very severe, cannot detect blood pressure

Wiwanitkit V, 2005.

It is evidenced by mildly and variably low factors II, V, VII, VIII, IX, X, and XII, and by mild to moderate increase of fibrin degradation products as well as low platelet count and fibrinogen [58]. At present, changes in platelet counts by interaction between virus and platelet are clearly shown [59-60]. Fortunately, the majority of patients have compensated consumptive coagulopathy that rarely requires treatment [59-60]. Bleeding is probably caused by platelet activation and endothelium capillary damage, and can be recovered with normal saline [59-60]. The rash of skin, or petechiae, epistaxis and gum bleeding are common in mild and moderately severe cases [61]. Recently, Putintseva et al. studied bone marrow specimens obtained from patients with dengue infection and they found hyperplasia of megakaryocytic in 60% [62]. They proposed that dengue fever virus caused a transitory modification in the regulation of thrombopoiesis that could be possibly a consequence of lymphoid damage extending the thrombocytopenic state and contributing to the appearance of hemorrhagic complications [62]. There are some recent interesting studies on platelet counts and clinical correlation in dengue fever virus infection. Chang et al. studied 15 cases of dengue fever and reported that all patients had varying degrees of hepatomegaly and pleural effusion pleural from thoracic x-rays accompanied by a rapid increase in the hematocrit of more than 20% and a fall in platelet count to less than 100,000/microliters [63]. George et al. reported a great variety of manifestations of hemorrhage in patients with dengue fever [61]. They noted that those manifestations were common in severe cases [61]. Tripathi et al. reported their experience in an outbreak in Delhi where mortality of infection dropped if the patients came early to hospital [64]. With regard to hematologic diagnostic markers, Narayanan et al. noted that there was no correlation between platelet count and bleeding in the infection [65]. Garcia et al. noted that the majority of patients with dengue fever had maximal thrombocytopenia in the fifth day after the beginning of constitutional symptoms [66]. Moreover, they identified the three phases: a) proteinuria and hypoalbuminemia; b) maximal cytopenia; and b) bradycardia and liver enzyme elevation, in the succession of events seen in the majority of patients with dengue fever that accompanied thrombocytopenia [66]. Finally, Gomber et al. reported that there is a poor association of thrombocytopenia with bleeding manifestation [67]. As previously mentioned, leukocyte disorder in patients with infection of dengue fever virus is described as lymphocytosis [7-8, 57]. Nevertheless, the average level of total white blood cell count is not high, and the range is wide. Therefore, implication directly to the infection is limited. Another observation is that the immune response of the host is an important factor in the course of illness [68]. The main response to this viral infection is lymphocytosis. Nevertheless, a mainly qualitative rather than a quantitative response might be more responsible for the host versus pathogen interaction mechanism of fever. Truly, at times those qualitative responses result in severe hypovolemic shock, known as DSS [69-70]. Nevertheless, it cannot be concluded that fever and "the disorder of leukocyte" are "without any relation", justified by the data showing absence of correlation since both fever and WBC changes could still related to a single process of pathophysiology (for example: the production of cytokine).

Concerning the hematocrit change, the hemoconcentration is another hallmark hematological manifestation in dengue infection. The leak of intravascular fluid is believed to be the main cause of the hemoconcentration in patients with dengue infections. However, Wiwanitkit and Manusvanich noted that hematocrit at admission of a dengue case might not be a useful parameter in prediction of the outcome of the patient [34]. This means that a hematocrit test on admission cannot predict shock in the hospitalized dengue hemorrhagic case [34]. In conclusion, hemoconcentration, lymphocytosis and decreased platelet are the three common hematological manifestations in patients with dengue infections.

In additional to hematological manifestation, uncommon clinical presentations of dengue infection are also documented. Hepatic manifestation is an interesting uncommon presentation of dengue infection. Indeed, hepatomegaly can be detected in the early stage of dengue infection (Table 2). The abnormality of liver function test is also reported. Recently, Rigau-Perez carried out a study that aimed at uncovering characteristics of DHF occurring in Puerto Rico [71]. In this work, Rigau-Perez found that high aspartate and alanine amino transferase (AST and ALT) levels were frequently found [71]. Mohan et al. carried out an interesting study to document abnormality of liver function in patients with dengue fever and found that levels of serum AST, ALT and alkaline phosphatase (ALP) on admission were raised in 80–87% of children with hepatomegaly, and 81% of cases without hepatomegaly [72]. They suggested a transitory inconvenience of liver functions in childhood, more common in DSS and DHF, with or without hepatomegaly [72]. According to these studies, aberrant result of liver function test seems not to be a rare presentation in the patients with the infection of dengue fever virus. In the most severe cases, liver failure is also reported [73]. The neurological manifestation is another rare presentation of dengue infection. In 2001, Pancharoen and Thisyakorn carried out a study to determine frequency and natural history of neurological manifestations of the infection of dengue fever virus in 1,493 Thai children [74]. They found that there were 80 children, classified in 20 cases of dengue fever, 26 cases of DHF and 34 cases of DSS, identifying with neurological manifestations, an incident of 5.4% of all patients of dengue infection [74]. All experienced the neurological manifestations during feverish phase of illness [74]. The patients were classified in a group of encephalitic (called dengue fever encephalopathy) (42), a seizure group (35) and a various group (3) [74]. The patients with encephalitic presented with modification of consciousness (83.3%), seizure (45.2%), confusion (23.8% mental), inflexibility (21.4%), spasticity (9.5%), clonus positive (4.8%), hemiplegia (2.4%) and kernig sign positive (2.4%), and they were older than those in the other groups [74]. The patients in the group of seizure presented with seizure (100%) and clonus positive (2.9%) [74]. The abnormal results of laboratory investigations included hyponatremia, abnormal enzymes of liver and pleocytosis of CSF [74]. The rate of general mortality was 5% [74]. Pancharoen and Thisyakorn concluded that the neurological manifestations including seizure and encephalopathy in children with fever were not rare while dengue fever encephalitis was rare [74].

Diagnosis of Dengue Infection

There are many present advances in the diagnosis of dengue fever [75]. Nevertheless, the majority of the diagnoses in the endemic area are generally based on medical history and basic investigation including the tourniquet test and platelet count. A positive tourniquet test is one of the various clinical parameters considered important by the World Health Organization in the diagnosis of DHF [76]. The tourniquet test is a useful test in investigation for infection of dengue fever virus. Recently, Cao et al. carried out an evaluation on the diagnostic property of this test for investigation for the infection of dengue fever virus in Vietnam [76]. In this study, a future evaluation of a classical test by sphygmomanometer, compared with a simple elastic tourniquet test, was carried out in 1,136 children with suspected infection of dengue fever virus [76]. According to this study, there was a good agreement among independent observers for both techniques, but the method of sphygmomanometer resulted in larger numbers of petechiae [76]. This classical method had a sensivity of 41.6% for the infection of dengue fever virus, with a specificity of 94.4%, positive predictive value of 98.3% and negative predictive value of 17.3%. Nevertheless, the test differentiated poorly among DHF (45% positive) and dengue fever (38% positive) [76]. Cao et al. concluded that conventional test added little in the diagnosis of dengue fever in hospitalized patients [76]. They also noted that a simple, cheap, and elastic turnstile might be useful in diagnosing infection of dengue fever virus in busy rural stations in the fever-endemic areas of the tropics [76]. Besides, they proposed that a positive test should incite close observation or early referring to hospital, but a negative test did not exclude the infection of dengue fever virus [76]. The hemaglutination inhibition, neutralization and assays of IgG ELISA are examples of routine investigation for confirmation of dengue fever virus infection. Guzman and Kouri noted that IgM ELISA, isolation of virus in mosquito cell lines and live mosquitoes, specific monoclonal antibodies and PCR represented great advances in the diagnosis of dengue fever [77]. Kowitdamrong et al. noted that discovery of HELLO titer was still useful for diagnosis, although coupled serum had to be taken [78].

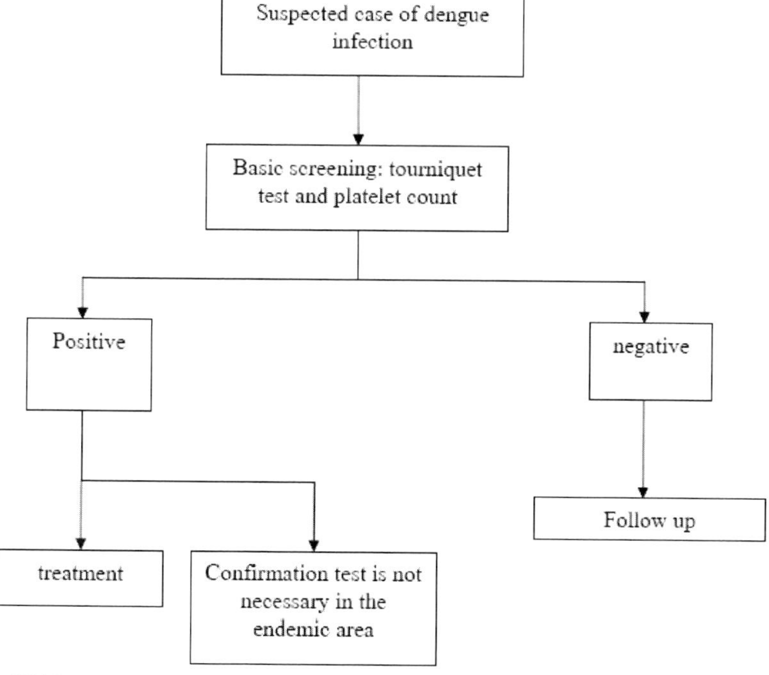

Wiwanitkit V, 2005.

Figure 3.1. Schematic diagram for diagnosis of dengue infection.

They noted that interval of time should be at least seven days for suspected primary infection, but a shorter interval could be considered for suspected secondary infection cases [78]. They also noted that exact and fast discovery of dengue fever IgM had become more useful because only single serum was required and an order for the dengue fever IgM test should be done after day 5 of the illness [78]. Nevertheless, Kowitdamrong et al. mentioned that interpretation of result should be carefully done according to the time of serum collection [78]. Schilling et al. studied sensivity of discovery of IgM antibody in coupled samples serum of 43 patients with or with primary or secondary dengue fever [79]. According to this study, samples of patients with primary dengue fever taken during days 1–3 of the illness displayed no IgM antibody [79]. During days 4–7 and after day 7, IgM antibody was discerned in 55% and 94%, respectively [79]. They noted that titers of IgG was significantly more high in the secondary dengue fever compared to those of primary dengue fever cases and high (>1280) titers was also found in some primary dengue fever patients [79]. Finally, Schilling et al. concluded an early diagnosis in numerous patients with acute dengue fever would be obtained only combining discovery of Ig M antibody with discovery of viral RNA or virus using RT-PCR [79].

Concerning the molecular diagnosis of dengue infection, there are several attempts to developed new molecular – based test for this purpose. However, most of the molecular diagnostic tools are considered expensive and not proper for the endemic area, which are usually poor and underprivileged. Guzman and Kouri said that an appropriate, fast, and accessible diagnosis test for epidemiological surveillance and clinical diagnosis was needed still [77]. Besides, they noted that tools that suggested a prognosis allowing for better management were also needed [77]. Finally, they proposed that infrastructure of laboratory and technical skill capacity should be improved in endemic countries in the order to influence positively dengue fever surveillance, clinical administration of infected case and development of new foci for control of dengue fever [77].

Pathology and Complication

A. Pathology

Several dengue pathologies are reported. The principal change is on the hematological system and endothelium, as previously mentioned. The platelet destruction, relating to immunopathology, is proposed. Nevertheless, preserved size of platelet is recently retrieved [80]. Furthermore, effusion collection in body cavities because of escape of intravascular fluid is noted. Histopathologically, generalized hemorrhage can be seen and hemorrhagic infarction of several visceral organs such as the stomach, lung and liver are noted. An et al. recently studied pathology of central nervous system in dengue infection in mice models [81]. According to this study, a high viral titer and antigens were detected in brain and vertebral rope after the inoculation [81]. To the first steps of infection, examinations of ultrastructures showed a few virions were present in the cytoplasm of ependymal cells lining the central canal [81]. As infection progress, virions were observed in the lumen of the rough endoplasmic reticulum (RER), RER-derived vesicles and the Golgi region of infected neuron

[81]. They suggested that dengue virus could spread to neuron of vertebral rope through cerebral spinal fluid and causes several pathologic neuronal responses [81]. Chen et al. executed another study on liver pathology in mice models with dengue infection [82]. According to this study, a strong correlation was found between activation of T cell and hepatic infiltration in immunocompetent infected mice infected with dengue virus [82]. They also noted for elevation of liver enzyme corresponded to activation of T cell [82]. Chen et al. suggested a relation between infiltration of T cell and elevation of liver enzymes [82]. About kidney pathology, infection of dengue is mentioned for its effect on kidney histopathologgy [83]. The change of glomeruli is noted in the patients with dengue [83]. Boonpucknavig et al. recently described their observations on glomerular pathology in 20 Thai dengue patients [84]. In this study, they executed percutaneous needle biopsies on the kidneys of 20 patients that had DHF with some clinical manifestation of kidney disturbances [84]. According to this study, IgG or IgM, or the two, and C3 could be localized in glomeruli, using the antibody fluorescent technique, in ten cases [84]. Electron microscopy showed focal basement membrane thickening of glomerulus, with hypertrophy of mesangial cells at sites where immunized complex was showed [84]. Furthermore, dense and spherical particles, 40 to 50 nm in the diameter, were found in 12 cases and these particles were carried in glomeruli by the monocyte-like cells [84].

B. Complications

Many complications of dengue infection have been documented in the medical literature. The most common complication in the infection of dengue virus is hemorrhagic episode. The hemorrhage can be found in a lot of organs included the retina [85]. Another serious common complication in dengue infection is shock. DSS is defined as a potentially mortal complication of this viral infection associated with hypotension and leakage of plasma into extravascular space. Bethell et al. studied microvascular permeability by the usage of gauge tension plethysmography in the Vietnamese children with DSS, or DHF without the shock, and in healthy children to determine if basic pathophysiology of DSS is distinct to less severe forms of disease [86]. They found that fluid resuscitation, the mean coefficient of microvascular permeability (K(f)) for the patients with dengue was approximately 50% higher than that for healthy control and there was not significant difference in K (f) between the two groups of patients, suggesting basic similar pathophysiology [86]. Bethell et al. puts a hypothesis that the variations in K (f) in the patients with DSS were bigger than those in the patients with DHF, which led to short-lived peaks of markedly increased permeability of microvascular components and consecutive hemodynamic shocks [86]. The other rare complications of dengue infection include the hepatitis [87], spleen rupture [88], rhabdomyolysis [89] and the syndrome of hemophagocytosis [90]. Souza et al. recently studied the hepatitis incidence in 1,585 dengue infected cases [87]. Among the 1,585 serologically confirmed cases of dengue, 44.5% presented high presented, with increased levels of at least one of the liver enzymes, 16.9% presented high aminotransferase, with levels of at least one of enzymes increased to more than three times above reference values and 3.8% of patients had progressed to the hepatic failure [87]. Souza et al. said that liver damage with elevation of aminotransferases and hepatic failure were a common complication of dengue infection [87]. Concerning spleen rupture, Imbert et al. said that this complication was rare, and examination of surgical specimen confirmed the organ to be softened and enlarged with formation of subcapsular hematoma [88]. Regarding rhabdomyolysis, Davis and Bourke noted that all patients with the viral infection must undergo urine analysis, and levels of serum creatinine kinase should be measured if the urine analysis revealed heme [89]. Regarding the syndrome of haemophagocytosis, Rueda et al. recommends that an aspiration of bone marrow should executed for differential diagnosis study in extended fever associated with dengue, as there was a possibility that this complication could be secondary haemophagocytic syndrome [90].

Treatment

Treatment of dengue infection should be based on the severity of the infection (Table 3). The concept of treatment is similar to other infections: getting rid of the pathogen or control of the infection and supportive or symptomatic treatment. In dengue infection, the specific antiviral drug for dengue virus is not available at present. There are some recent reports on the possible antiviral drugs for dengue virus infection. Damonte et al. recently noted that various alga sulfated polysaccharides showed high antiviral activity against dengue virus and these polysaccharides should be further studied aiming at drug development [91]. Crance et al. recently evaluated antiviral activities of ribavirin, interferon-alpha (IFN-ALPHA), azauridine and glycyrrhizin against 11 flaviviruses pathogenic including dengue fever [92]. They found that ribavirin and of azauridine resulted assets in replica of tested pathogenic flaviviruses in the concentrations that did not alter normal morphology of cell, but they were not selective inhibitors when selectivity were evaluated with regard to the inhibition of growth of cell on account of cytostatic effect while glycyrrhizin inhibited replica of flaviviruses in higher concentrations [92]. Crance et al. concluded that these precincts of antiflavivirus should be further evaluated for their efficacy in treatment of infections of flavivirus in vivo [92]. With respect to supporting treatment, correction of vascular collapse should be main consideration. In grade I or II of dengue fever, blood pressures of patients do not yet seriously diminish and extensive liquid replacement is not necessary. Oral liquid replacement is sufficient for these cases. The hospitalization in these cases is not necessary. To descend fever, paracetamol should be utilized. It should be noted that aspirin is contraindicated in these cases. A complication due to additional disturbance of platelet according to utilization of salicylate in dengue infection is extensively mentioned. Following up of patients with grade I or II of dengue fever should be put in 1 week according to course of viral illness. It should be noted that phase of the illness can change higher, therefore, suggestion for patients to observe their symptoms and to visit physician again if the symptoms get worse are indicated.

In the severe case of dengue infection (grade III or IV), fluid replacement should be considered with care. Hospitalization is required. The intravenous liquid replacement is indicated for all cases. The ideal fluid for administration should include cystalloids or colloids (including albumen) [93]. Cystalloids is given like alimentary boluses as quickly as possible, and so much as two to three alimentary boluses are needed in deep shock [93]. The colloidal liquids are indicated in patients with massive shrinkage of plasma and in whom a large volume of cystalloids has been given [93]. Soni et al. noted that key for success in taking care of severe dengue fever patients were frequent control of patients and changing strategies corresponding to the clinical change [93]. They noted that an ascent in hematocrit of 20% along with a continuous drop of platelet count was an important indicator for beginning of shock [93]. Aside from correction of electrolyte and metabolic disturbances, oxygen is obligatory in all patients with shock [93]. Besides, some patients develop DIC and they need supporting therapy with products of blood (blood, FFP and platelet) [93]. With respect to fluid replacement in severe cases of dengue fever with shock, Excrement et al. said that Dextran 70 provided the fastest normalization of the hematocrit and restoration of cardiac index, without adverse effects, and they can be preferred solution for acute resuscitation in DSS [94]. Ngo et al. recently carried out a relative study in 4 fluid replacement regimens for severe dengue fever [95]. They undertook a blinded randomized comparison of 4 liquids (dextran, gelatin, lactated Ringer's, and normal saline) for initial resuscitation of 230 Vietnamese children with DSS [95]. In this study, all children survived, and there was no difference in advantage on using any of the 4 liquids, but the most long times of the recovery occurred in lactated Ringer's [95]. As guideline for general practitioner, the author proposed the beginning of intravenous liquid replacement with 0,9% normal saline solution at the rate of 20 Ml/kg/hour in the first 2 hours then continue for 10 Ml/kg/hour for the next 6 hours then left the fluid for to be instilled within the next 16 hours. The response of fluid replacement can be monitored from serial taking of blood pressure and manual hematocrit test. It should be noted that the fluid replacement should not exceed 24 hour to avoid the redistribution of liquid and possible liquid drunkenness in convalescent phase. The intravenous administration of corticosteroid is not contraindicated and shown to be useful in some cases [96 - 97].

Prevention

The prevention of dengue infection key in controlling this viral disease. Since this disease is spread by vector-borne transmission, the control of the vector is important in primary prevention. In order to control the mosquito, the use of bed nets and pesticides should be considered. However, the application of vector-control methods are labor intensive, require discipline and diligence, and are hard to sustain [98].

More details will be presented in the final chapter. An advance in the prevention of dengue infection is the attempt to develop a vaccine for this disease.

Concerning vaccination for dengue, there are many interesting recent reports on this topic. Pang noted that various promising candidates of vaccine in the form of live, reduced and chimerical vaccines had been developed and they were at present in the human clinical trial phase [99]. The polyvalent vaccines of dengue fever are now in late development and are an extraordinary challenge regarding security of the vaccine, in which primary or secondary failures of the vaccine might give rise to antibody-dependent enhanced (ADE) wild-type dengue infections [100]. For example, in 2004, Blaney et al. reported that during their experiment, the rDEN3/4(ME) and rDEN3/4Delta30(ME) antigenic chimerical virus could be considered for evaluation in humans and for inclusion in a tetravalent dengue vaccine [101]. Nevertheless, scientific, logistic, practical, and significant challenges remain before these vaccines can be responsibly and extensively applied to vulnerable populations [99]. Baize et al. said that a focus of the vaccine against dengue fever was possible and should induce stable immune responses with cell and humoral components, and should avoid potential deleterious effects that are associated with such immune responses [102]. Pang said that control of the vector, education of the community and sanitary measures should continue in parallel with development of a vaccine [99].

References

[1] Mairuhu AT, Wagenaar J, Brandjes DP, van Gorp EC. Dengue: an arthropod-borne disease of global importance. *Eur. J. Clin. Microbiol. Infect. Dis.* 23, 425-33 (2004)

[2] Nogueira SA. Dengue. *J. Pediatr. (Rio J).* 75(Suppl 1), S9-S14 (1999)

[3] Halstead SB. Dengue. *Curr. Opin. Infec.t Dis.* 15, 471-6 (2002)

[4] Jacobs M, Young P. Dengue vaccines: preparing to roll back dengue. *Curr. Opin, Investig, Drugs.* 4, 168-71 (2003)

[5] Wilson ME. The traveller and emerging infections: sentinel, courier, transmitter. *J. Appl. Microbiol.* 94 Suppl,1S-11S (2003)

[6] Malavige GN, Fernando S, Fernando DJ, Seneviratne SL. Dengue viral infections. *Postgrad. Med. J.* 80,588-601 (2004)

[7] Guzman MG, Kouri G. Dengue and dengue hemorrhagic fever in the Americas: lessons and challenges. *J. Clin. Virol.* 27, 1-13 (2003)

[8] Guzman MG, Kouri G. Dengue: an update. *Lancet. Infect. Dis.* 2, 33-42 (2002)

[9] Menard B. Geographic changes in exposure to dengue. *Sante.* 13, 89-94 (2003)

[10] Corwin AL, Larasati RP, Bangs MJ, Wuryadi S, Arjoso S, Sukri N, Listyaningsih E, Hartati S, Namursa R, Anwar Z, Chandra S, Loho B, Ahmad H, Campbell JR, Porter KR. Epidemic dengue transmission in southern Sumatra, Indonesia. *Trans. R. Soc. Trop. Med. Hyg.* 95, 257-65 (2001)

[11] Tuntaprasart W, Barbazan P, Nitatpattana N, Rongsriyam Y, Yoksan S, Gonzalez JP. Seroepidemiological survey among schoolchildren during the 2000-2001 dengue outbreak of Ratchaburi Province, Thailand. *Southeast. Asian. J. Trop. Med. Public. Health.* 34, 564-8 (2003)

[12] Pinheiro FP, Corber SJ. Global situation of dengue and dengue haemorrhagic fever, and its emergence in the Americas. *World. Health. Stat. Q.* 50, 161-9 (1997)

[13] Shah I, Deshpande GC, Tardeja PN. Outbreak of dengue in Mumbai and predictive markers for dengue shock syndrome. *J. Trop. Pediatr.* 50, 301-5 (2004)

[14] Arunachalam N, Murty US, Kabilan L, Balasubramanian A, Thenmozhi V, Narahari D, Ravi A, Satyanarayana K. Studies on dengue in rural areas of Kurnool District, Andhra Pradesh, India. *Am. Mosq. Control. Assoc.* 20, 87-90 (2004)

[15] Zhoa Z. Current status in the prevention and control of dengue fever in China.*Zhonghua. Liu. Xing. Bing. Xue. Za. Zhi.* 21, 223-4 (2000)

[16] Luo H, He J, Zheng K, Li L, Jiang L. Analysis on the epidemiologic features of Dengue fever in Guangdong province, 1990-2000. *Zhonghua. Liu. Xing. Bing. Xue. Za. Zhi.* 23, 427-30 (2002)

[17] DeHart RL. Health issues of air travel. *Annu. Rev. Public Health.* 2003;24:133-51 (2003)

[18] Reiskind MH, Baisley KJ, Calampa C, Sharp TW, Watts DM, Wilson ML. Epidemiological and ecological characteristics of past dengue virus infection in Santa Clara, Peru. *Trop. Med. Int. Health.* 6, 212-8 (2001)

[19] Vaughn DW. Invited commentary: Dengue lessons from Cuba. *Am. J. Epidemiol.* 152, 800-3 (2000)

[20] Haas W, Krause G, Marcus U, Stark K, Ammon A, Burger R. Emerging infectious diseases". Dengue-fever, West-Nile-fever, SARS, avian influenza, HIV. *Internist. (Berl).* 45, 684-92 (2004)

[21] Badiaga S, Barrau K, Brouqui P, Durant J, Malvy D, Janbon F, Bonnet E, Bosseray A, Sotto A, Peyramont D, Dydymski S, Cazorla C, Tolou H, Durant JP, Delmont J; Infectio-Sud Group. Imported Dengue in French University Hospitals: a 6-year survey. *J. Travel. Med.* 10, 286-9 (2003)

[22] Gascon J, Giner V, Vidal J, Jou JM, Mas E, Corachan M. Dengue: a re-emerging disease. A clinical and epidemiological study in 57 Spanish travelers. *Med. Clin. (Barc).* 111, 583-6 (1998)

[23] Fagbami AH, Monath TP, Fabiyi A. Dengue virus infections in Nigeria: a survey for antibodies in monkeys and humans. *Trans. R. Soc. Trop. Med. Hyg.* 71, 60-5 (1977)

[24] Gubler DJ, Sather GE, Kuno G, Cabral JR. Dengue 3 virus transmission in Africa. *Am. J. Trop. Med. Hyg.* 35, 1280-4 (1986)

[25] Rodier GR, Parra JP, Kamil M, Chakib SO, Cope SE. Recurrence and emergence of infectious diseases in Djibouti city. *Bull. World. Health. Organ.* 73, 755-9 (1995)

[26] Currie BJ, Brewster DR. Childhood infections in the tropical north of Australia. *J Paediatr .Child. Health.* 37, 326-30 (2001)

[27] Russell RC, Dwyer DE. Arboviruses associated with human disease in Australia. *Microbes. Infect.* 2,:1693-704 (2000)

[28] Malcolm RL, Hanna JN, Phillips DA. The timeliness of notification of clinically suspected cases of dengue imported into north Queensland. *Aust. N. Z. J. Public. Health.* 23, 414-7 (1999)

[29] Hills SL, Piispanen JP, Humphreys JL, Foley PN. A focal, rapidly-controlled outbreak of dengue fever in two suburbs in Townsville, north Queensland, 2001. *Commun. Dis. Intell.* 26, 596-600 (2001)

[30] Nogueira SA. Dengue. *J. Pediatr. (Rio J).* 75(Suppl 1), S9-S14 (1999)

[31] Rehle TM. Classification, distribution and importance of arboviruses. *Trop. Med. Parasitol.* 40, 391-5 (1989)

[32] Degallier N, Herve JP, Travassos da Rosa AP, Sa GC. Aedes aegypti (L.): importance of its bioecology in the transmission of dengue and other arboviruses. I. *Bull. Soc. Pathol. Exot. Filiales.* 81, 97-110 (1988)

[33] Thaithumyanon P, Thisyakorn U, Deerojnawong J, Innis BL. Dengue infection complicated by severe hemorrhage and vertical transmission in a parturient woman. *Clin. Infect. Dis.* 18, 248-9 (1994)

[34] Wiwanitkit V, Manusvanich P. Can hematocrit and platelet determination on admission predict shock in hospitalized children with dengue hemorrhagic fever? A clinical observation from a small outbreak. *Clin. Appl. Thromb. Hemost.* 10, 65-7 (2004)

[35] Ahmed S. Vertical transmission of dengue: first case report from Bangladesh. *Southeast. Asian. J. Trop. Med. Public. Health.* 34, 800-3 (2003)

[36] Chye JK, Lim CT, Ng KB, Lim JM, George R, Lam SK. Vertical transmission of dengue. *Clin. Infect. Dis.* 25, 1374-7 (1997)

[37] Failloux AB, Vazeille-Falcoz M, Mousson L, Rodhain F. Genetic control of vectorial competence in Aedes mosquitoes. *Bull. Soc. Pathol. Exot.* 92, 266-73 (1999)

[38] Failloux AB, Darius H, Pasteur N. Genetic differentiation of Aedes aegypti, the vector of dengue virus in French Polynesia. *J. Am. Mosq. Control. Assoc.* 11, 457-62 (1995)

[39] Gorrochotegui-Escalante N, Munoz ML, Fernandez-Salas I, Beaty BJ, Black WC 4th. Genetic isolation by distance among Aedes aegypti populations along the northeastern coast of Mexico. *Am. J. Trop. Med. Hyg.* 62, 200-9 (2000)

[40] Tran KT, Vazeille-Falcoz M, Mousson L, Tran HH, Rodhain F, Ngugen TH, Failloux AB. Aedes aegypti in Ho Chi Minh City (Viet Nam): susceptibility to dengue 2 virus and genetic differentiation. *Trans. R. Soc. Trop. Med. Hyg.* 93, 581-6 (1999)

[41] Fernandez-Mestre MT, Gendzekhadze K, Rivas-Vetencourt P, Layrisse Z. TNF-alpha-308A allele, a possible severity risk factor of hemorrhagic manifestation in dengue fever patients. *Tissue. Antigens.* 64, 469-72 (2004)

[42] Loke H, Bethell D, Phuong CX, Day N, White N, Farrar J, Hill A. Susceptibility to dengue hemorrhagic fever in vietnam: evidence of an association with variation in the vitamin d receptor and Fc gamma receptor IIa genes. *Am. J. Trop. Med. Hyg.* 67, 102-6 (2002)

[43] Martinez-Torres E. Dengue and hemorrhagic dengue: the clinical aspects. *Salud. Publica. Mex.* 37 Suppl, S29-44 (1995)

[44] Hayes EB, Gubler DJ. Dengue and dengue hemorrhagic fever. *Pediatr. Infect. Dis. J.* 11, 311-7 (1992)

[45] Courageot MP, Catteau A, Despres P. Mechanisms of dengue virus-induced cell death. *Adv. Virus. Res.* 60, 57-86 (2003)

[46] Mitrakul C. Bleeding problem in dengue haemorrhagic fever: platelets and coagulation changes. *Southeast. Asian. J. Trop. Med. Public. Health.* 18, 407-12 (1987)

[47] Falconar AK. dengue virus nonstructural-1 protein (NS1) generates antibodies to common epitopes on human blood clotting, integrin/adhesin proteins and binds to human endothelial cells: potential implications in haemorrhagic fever pathogenesis. *Arch. Virol.* 142, 897-916 (1997)

[48] Wang S, He R, Patarapotikul J, Innis BL, Anderson R. Antibody-enhanced binding of dengue-2 virus to human platelets. *Virology* 213, 254-7 (1995)

[49] Wiwanitkit V. Dengue virus nonstructural-1 protein and its phylogenetic correlation to human fibrinogen and thrombocytes: a study to explain hemorrhagic complication. *Int J Genom Proteom* 1, 2 (2004)

[50] Chang HH, Shyu HF, Wang YM, Sun DS, Shyu RH, Tang SS, Huang YS. Facilitation of cell adhesion by immobilized dengue viral nonstructural protein 1 (NS1): arginine-glycine-aspartic acid structural mimicry within the dengue viral NS1 antigen. *J. Infect. Dis.* 186, 743-51 (2002)

[51] Wiwanitkit V. Platelet CD61 might play an important role in causing hemorrhagic complication in dengue infection. *Clin. Appl. Thrombo. Hemostat.* 11, 112 (2005)

[52] Lei HY, Yeh TM, Liu HS, Lin YS, Chen SH, Liu CC. Immunopathogenesis of dengue virus infection. *J. Biomed. Sci.* 8, 377-88 (2001)

[53] Rodriguez-Ortega M. Nitric oxide in dengue pathology. *Acta. Cient. Venez.* 49 Suppl 1, 8-12 (1998)

[54] da Fonseca BA, Fonseca SN. Dengue virus infections. *Curr. Opin. Pediatr.* 14, 67-71 (2002)

[55] Wiwanitkit V. Bleeding and other presentations in Thai patients with dengue infection. *Clin. Appl. Thromb. Hemost.* 10, 397-8 (2004)

[56] Aggarwal A, Chandra J, Aneja S, Patwari AK, Dutta AK. An epidemic of dengue hemorrhagic fever and dengue shock syndrome in children in Delhi. *Indian. Pediatr.* 35, 727-32 (1998)

[57] Solomon T, Mallewa M. Dengue and other emerging flaviviruses. *J. Infect.* 42, 104-15 (2001)

[58] Mitrakul C, Poshyachinda M, Futrakul P, Sangkawibha N, Ahandrik S. Hemostatic and platelet kinetic studies in dengue hemorrhagic fever. *Am. J. Trop. Med. Hyg.* 26, 975-84 (1977)

[59] Halstead SB. Dengue. *Curr. Opin. Infect. Dis.* 15, 471-6 (2002)

[60] Almagro Vazquez D, Gonzalez Cabrera I, Cruz Gomez Y, Castaneda Morales M. Platelet function in dengue hemorrhagic fever. *Acta. Haematol.* 70, 276-7 (1983)

[61] George R, Duraisamy G. Bleeding manifestations of dengue haemorrhagic fever in Malaysia. *Acta. Trop.* 38, 71-8 (1981)

[62] Putintseva E, Vega G, Fernandez L. Alterations in thrombopoiesis in patients with thrombocytopenia produced by dengue hemorrhagic fever. *Nouv. Rev. Fr. Hematol.* 28, 269-73 (1986)

[63] Chang CS, Harn MR, Nimmannitya S. Clinical observation of 15 Thai children with dengue hemorrhagic fever. *Gaoxiong. Yi. Xue. Ke. Xue. Za. Zhi.* 6, 131-6 (1990)

[64] Tripathi BK, Gupta B, Sinha RS, Prasad S, Sharma DK. Experience in adult population in dengue outbreak in Delhi. *J. Assoc. Physicians. India.* 46, 273-6 (1998)

[65] Narayanan M, Aravind MA, Thilothammal N, Prema R, Sargunam CS, Ramamurty N. Dengue fever epidemic in Chennai--a study of clinical profile and outcome. *Indian. Pediatr.* 39,1027-33 (2002)

[66] Garcia S, Morales R, Hunter RF. Dengue fever with thrombocytopenia: studies towards defining vulnerability of bleeding. *Bol. Asoc. Med. P. R.* 87, 2-7 (1995)

[67] Gomber S, Ramachandran VG, Kumar S, Agarwal KN, Gupta P, Gupta P, Dewan DK. Hematological observations as diagnostic markers in dengue hemorrhagic fever--a reappraisal. *Indian. Pediatr.* 38, 477-81 (2001)

[68] Vaughn DW, Green S, Kalayanarooj S, Innis BL, Nimmannitya S, Suntayakorn S, Endy TP, Raengsakulrach B, Rothman AL, Ennis FA, Nisalak A. Dengue viremia titer,

antibody response pattern, and virus serotype correlate with disease severity. *J. Infect. Dis.* 181, 2-9 (2000)

[69] Srichaikul T, Nimmannitya S. Haematology in dengue and dengue haemorrhagic fever. *Baillieres. Best. Pract. Res. Clin. Haematol.* 13, 261-76 (2000)

[70] Bhamarapravati N. Hemostatic defects in dengue hemorrhagic fever. *Rev. Infect. Dis.* 11 Suppl 4, S826-9 (1989)

[71] Rigau-Perez JG. Clinical manifestations of dengue hemorrhagic fever in Puerto Rico, 1990-1991. Puerto Rico Association of Epidemiologists. *Rev. Panam. Salud. Publica.* 1, 381-8 (1997)

[72] Mohan B, Patwari AK, Anand VK. Hepatic dysfunction in childhood dengue infection. *J. Trop. Pediatr.* 46, 40-3 (2000)

[73] Lawn SD, Tilley R, Lloyd G, Finlayson C, Tolley H, Newman P, Rice P, Harrison TS. Dengue hemorrhagic fever with fulminant hepatic failure in an immigrant returning to Bangladesh. *Clin. Infect. Dis.* 37, e1-4 (2003)

[74] Pancharoen C, Thisyakorn U. Neurological manifestations in dengue patients. *Southeast. Asian. J. Trop. Med. Public. Health.* 32, 341-5 (2001)

[75] Shu PY, Huang JH. Current advances in dengue diagnosis. *Clin. Diagn. Lab. Immunol.* 11, 642-50 (2004)

[76] Cao XT, Ngo TN, Wills B, Kneen R, Nguyen TT, Ta TT, Tran TT, Doan TK, Solomon T, Simpson JA, White NJ, Farrar JJ; Dong Nai Paediatric Hospital Study Group. Evaluation of the World Health Organization standard tourniquet test and a modified tourniquet test in the diagnosis of dengue infection in Viet Nam. *Trop. Med. Int. Health.* 7, 125-32 (2002)

[77] Guzman MG, Kouri G. Dengue diagnosis, advances and challenges. *Int J Infect Dis. 2004* Mar;8(2):69-80 (2004)

[78] Kowitdamrong E, Thammaborvorn R, Semboonlor L, Mungmee V, Bhattarakosol P. Detection of dengue HI and IgM antibody: is it diagnostically useful? when and how? *J. Med. Assoc. Thai.* 84 Suppl 1, S148-54 (2001)

[79] Schilling S, Ludolfs D, Van An L, Schmitz H. Laboratory diagnosis of primary and secondary dengue infection. *J. Clin. Virol.* 2004 Nov;31(3):179-84.(2004)

[80] Wiwanitkit V. Mean platelet volume in the patients with dengue hemorrhagic fever. *Platelets.* 15, 185 (2004)

[81] An J, Zhou DS, Kawasaki K, Yasui K. The pathogenesis of spinal cord involvement in dengue virus infection. *Virchows. Arch.* 442, 472-81 (2003)

[82] Chen HC, Lai SY, Sung JM, Lee SH, Lin YC, Wang WK, Chen YC, Kao CL, King CC, Wu-Hsieh BA. Lymphocyte activation and hepatic cellular infiltration in immunocompetent mice infected by dengue virus. *J. Med. Virol.* 73, 419-31 (2004)

[83] Boonpucknavig V, Soontornniyomkij V. Pathology of renal diseases in the tropics. *Semin. Nephrol.* 23, 88-106 (2003)

[84] Boonpucknavig V, Bhamarapravati N, Boonpucknavig S, Futrakul P, Tanpaichitr P. Glomerular changes in dengue hemorrhagic fever. *Arch. Pathol. Lab. Med.* 100, 206-12 (1976)

[85] Spitznas M. Macular haemorrhage in dengue fever (author's transl). *Klin. Monatsbl. Augenheilkd.* 172, 105-7 (1978)

[86] Bethell DB, Gamble J, Pham PL, Nguyen MD, Tran TH, Ha TH, Tran TN, Dong TH, Gartside IB, White NJ, Day NP. Noninvasive measurement of microvascular leakage in patients with dengue hemorrhagic fever. *Clin. Infect. Dis.* 32, 243-53 (2001)

[87] Souza LJ, Alves JG, Nogueira RM, Gicovate Neto C, Bastos DA, Siqueira EW, Souto Filho JT, Cezario Tde A, Soares CE, Carneiro Rda C. Aminotransferase changes and acute hepatitis in patients with dengue fever: analysis of 1,585 cases. *Braz. J. Infect. Dis.* 8, 156-63 (2004)

[88] Imbert P, Sordet D, Hovette P, Touze JE. Spleen rupture in a patient with dengue fever. *Trop. Med. Parasitol.* 44, 327-8 (1993)

[89] Davis JS, Bourke P. Rhabdomyolysis associated with dengue virus infection. *Clin. Infect. Dis.* 38, e109-11(2004)

[90] Rueda E, Mendez A, Gonzalez G. Hemophagocytic syndrome associated with dengue hemorrhagic fever. *Biomedica.* 22, 160-6 (2002)

[91] Damonte EB, Matulewicz MC, Cerezo AS. Sulfated seaweed polysaccharides as antiviral agents. *Curr. Med. Chem.* 11, 2399-419 (2004)

[92] Crance JM, Scaramozzino N, Jouan A, Garin D. Interferon, ribavirin, 6-azauridine and glycyrrhizin: antiviral compounds active against pathogenic flaviviruses. *Antiviral. Res.* 58, 73-9 (2003)

[93] Soni A, Chugh K, Sachdev A, Gupta D. Management of dengue fever in ICU. *Indian. J. Pediatr.* 68, 1051-5 (2001)

[94] Dung NM, Day NP, Tam DT, Loan HT, Chau HT, Minh LN, Diet TV, Bethell DB, Kneen R, Hien TT, White NJ, Farrar JJ. Fluid replacement in dengue shock syndrome: a randomized, double-blind comparison of four intravenous-fluid regimens. *Clin. Infect. Dis.* 29, 787-94 (1999)

[95] Ngo NT, Cao XT, Kneen R, Wills B, Nguyen VM, Nguyen TQ, Chu VT, Nguyen TT, Simpson JA, Solomon T, White NJ, Farrar J. Acute management of dengue shock syndrome: a randomized double-blind comparison of 4 intravenous fluid regimens in the first hour. *Clin. Infect. Dis.* 32, 204-13 (2001)

[96] Sumarmo, Talogo W, Asrin A, Isnuhandojo B, Sahudi A. Failure of hydrocortisone to affect outcome in dengue shock syndrome. *Pediatrics.* 69, 45-9 (1982)

[97] Tassniyom S, Vasanawathana S, Chirawatkul A, Rojanasuphot S. Failure of high-dose methylprednisolone in established dengue shock syndrome: a placebo-controlled, double-blind study. *Pediatrics.* 92, 111-5 (1993)

[98] Guzman MG, Mune M, Kouri G. Dengue vaccine: priorities and progress. *Expert Rev. Anti. Infect. Ther.* 2, 895-911 (2004)

[99] Pang T. Vaccines for the prevention of neglected diseases--dengue fever. *Curr. Opin. Biotechnol.* 14, 332-6 (2003)

[100] Halstead SB, Heinz FX, Barrett AD, Roehrig JT. Dengue virus: molecular basis of cell entry and pathogenesis, 25-27 June 2003, Vienna, Austria. *Vaccine.* 23, 849-56 (2005)

[101] Blaney JE Jr, Hanson CT, Firestone CY, Hanley KA, Murphy BR, Whitehead SS.Genetically modified, live attenuated dengue virus type 3 vaccine candidates. *Am. J. Trop. Med. Hyg.* 71, 811-21 (2004)

[102] Baize S, Marianneau P, Georges-Courbot MC, Deubel V. Recent advances in vaccines against viral haemorrhagic fevers. *Curr. Opin. Infect. Dis.* 14, 513-8(2001)

Chapter V

Yellow Fever

Introduction to Yellow Fever

Yellow fever is an infection carried by mosquitoes. This is a contagious disease caused by an arbovirus, the yellow fever virus [1]. The agent is maintained in the cycles of jungle primates as the vertebrate hosts and the mosquitoes, especially *Aedes* in Africa, and *Haemagogus* and *Sabethes* in America [1]. It is transmitted in a cycle implying monkeys and mosquitoes, but the human can also serve as host of viremia for the mosquito infection [2]. Today, the disease affects as many as 200,000 people yearly in the tropical regions. Africa and South America report a significant danger to non-vaccinated travelers to these sectors [2]. Approximately 90% of the infections are soft, or asymptomatic, while 10% are clinically severe with a 50% death rate [1]. This disease can be classified as an original viral hemorrhagic, similar to the fever of dengue and the infection of Chikungunya. Yellow fever is principally distributed in Africa, where the urban epidemics are on the rise [1]. The disease is diagnosed by serology (the detection of IgM), virus isolation, immunohistochemistry and the RT-PCR [1].

Yellow fever is a zoonosis and cannot be eliminated, but it is avoidable in humans while using the specific vaccine [1]. Monath reported that the disease's mechanisms were poorly understood and had not been the focus of research in modern medicine [2]. Monath noted that yellow fever was one of the more feared deadly diseases before the development of an effective vaccine [2]. Monath also mentioned that since there was no specific treatment and direction of patients with the disease was extremely problematic, the accent was on the preventive vaccination [2]. A dose should protect an individual for at least 10 years, after which revaccination is recommended [1]. The new applications using yellow fever 17D viruses as a vector for the foreign genes holds considerable promise as a means of developing a vaccine against the other viruses, and probably against cancers [2].

Although there was much effort over decades in getting rid of this disease, the infection always sporadically arrives. As a zoonosis, yellow fever cannot be eliminated, but the reduction of the disease burden can be possible by implementing a routine practice of childhood vaccination in the endemic countries, which is inexpensive when the advantages are taken into account [2]. According to the globalization at this moment, the yellow fever has emerged as a contagious problem not only in tropical but also in nontropical countries. The vaccination for the traveler is proposed for the yellow fever [3-5]. The knowledge of yellow fever is, therefore, an interesting subject for non-specialized doctors all over the world.

Worldwide Epidemiology of Yellow Fever

Recent increases in the density and distribution of the urban mosquito vector, *Aedes aegypti*, as well as an increase in airplane travel, have led to an increase in the risk of introduction and extension of the yellow fever to North and Central America, the Caribbean and Asia [2]. In South America, in the years 1970–2001, 4,543 cases were reported in many parts of Peru (51.5%), Bolivia (20.1%) and Brazil (18.7%) [1]. Recently, Gubler noted that yellow fever was an old illness, causing the greater epidemics in past centuries [6]. Gubler noted that the illness was well controlled in the 1900s, yellow fever in French-speaking Africa by vaccination and yellow fever in the Americas by effective control of the main urban vector of the virus, *Aedes aegypti*. Nevertheless, Gubler noted that there was a resurgence of yellow fever in Africa in the last 25 years of the 20th century [6]. Barrett and Monath recently mentioned the correlation between a change in the epidemiology and a change in the ecology of yellow fever virus [7]. A summary of some recent reports on the epidemiology of yellow fever in several regions of the world is presented.

A. Africa

Africa is an endemic area very well acquainted with yellow fever. The World Health Organization estimates that there are 200,000 cases including 30,000 deaths, and 90% occur in Africa [8-9]. Mutebi and Barrett noted that yellow fever was still a greater public problem, especially in Africa, in spite of the availability of a very efficient vaccine [8]. Tomori noted that yellow fever reappears with vehemence, to constitute a greater sanitary problem in Africa in the last two decades, and that this illness had brought unheard-of difficulty and indescribable misery among different populations in Africa [9]. Tomori also said that yellow fever was one of Africa's barriers to social and economic development [9]. Between 1939 and 1952, the yellow fever virtually disappeared in parts of Africa, where a systematic massive program of vaccination was in place [9]. Mutebi and Barrett noted that the number of yellow fever cases has grown tremendously, with most yellow fever activity in Western Africa in the past two decades, and this increase in yellow fever activity was in part due to damage in the yellow fever vaccination and the mosquito controls programs [8].

Five viral genotypes of yellow fever were found in Africa, and every genotype circulates in a geographic distinct region [8]. West Africa genotype I, found in Nigeria and the surrounding sectors, is associated with frequent epidemics, while the three genotypes in the eastern and central regions of Africa are in the regions where the eruptions of yellow fever are rare [8]. Mutebi and Barrett said that the other factors, including the genetic and behavioral variation among the vector type, were also thought to play a role in the epidemiology of yellow fever in Africa [8]. The recent epidemics of yellow fever in Africa affected in a predominant way children under the age of 15 years [9]. Sang and Dungster noted that there was an increase in the frequency of eruptions, and the detection of arbovirus activities in humans and vectors in the last decade included the reappearance of yellow fever virus as a health worry for the public in Kenya [10]. They noted that recognition of importance of cases and diagnosis was critical to the direction and the surveillance [9]. Onyango et al. reported a recent eruption of fatal hemorrhagic fever, caused by the yellow fever virus that arrived in southern Soudan [11]. In this report, the analysis of phylogenetics showed that the virus belonged to the Eastern African genotype, which supported the dispute that yellow fever was endemic in Eastern Africa with the potential to cause major eruptions in humans [11]. Tomori noted that the reemergence of fever yellow in Africa and the failure to check the disease had resulted from a combination of several factors, including the following: a collapse of delivery systems of health care; the lack of recognition of the impact of the disease on the social and economical development of the affected communities; the insufficient political engagement in the surveillance by the governments of endemic countries; poor or inadequate disease supervision; the measures of check of inopportune diseases; and the avoidable poverty coupled with the misled priorities in resource benefits [9]. Finally, Tomori concluded that yellow fever can be kept in check in Africa during the next decade if the African governments seize the initiative for surveillance while declaring a resolution to control the disease, backed up with engagement and a sufficient budget which could lead to improved surveillance activities of yellow fever [9].

B. Asia

Although the infection of dengue virus—which has a mosquito vector similar to yellow fever—is common in Asia, yellow fever is not common in Asia. Despite the conditions in Asia that are favorable for the transmission of yellow fever, no information regarding eruption has been retrieved. In the past, yellow fever was reported as an important public health problem in South Asia [12]. A possible explanation is that a preceding infection with another flavivirus, especially the virus of dengue, can provide protection from yellow fever infection. Nevertheless, yellow fever has been noted as a new infection to emerge as a possible contagious disease in India for the past few years [13-14]. The supervision and surveillance of yellow fever are recommended [13-14]. In fact, eruptions of yellow fever in the regions where it had been absent is noted [15]. The change in the ecology is reported as an important factor [12, 15]. Furthermore, Tomori recently mentioned the possible spreading of yellow fever in Asia and Oceania because of an increase in air travel among the endemic sector [16].

C. North America

North America is not considered an endemic sector of yellow fever. The slaves of Dutch merchants brought yellow fever from Africa to the Americas during the mid-seventeenth century [17]. For the next two and a half centuries, the disease terrorized maritime harbors throughout the Americas [17]. Through the nineteenth century, yellow fever was the blight of southern coastal cities [18]. Nevertheless, Tomori noted that the recent increases in density and the distribution of the mosquito vector, *Aedes aegypti*, just like the urban ascension in the air travel, increased the introduction risk and and spread of yellow fever to North America [16]. Tellow fever became an emerging important imported infection in the United States in the past few years. In fact, urban yellow fever was eliminated in the first half of this century, with the eradication of the mosquito vector in South America; nevertheless, the reinfestation that began in the 1970s is now almost complete, and the vector surveillance is considerably more difficult now than before [19]. Tomori mentioned that the urban yellow fever threat is greater in cities such as Santa Cruz, Bolivia, because of the proximity of the forest, but the improved transportation links increased the spreading probability by the viremic people to the sectors of non-endemicity [19]. Tomir also mentioned that since the inhabitants of the cities and many visited sectors in south coastal America had never been vaccinated, an eruption would facilitate over spreading of the disease, even to the other continents [19]. Tomori concluded that laboratory-based supervision, together with obstacle strategies and checks, are defensive measures against the future possible threat of urban epidemics [19].

D. Latin America and South America

There have been many recent reports on the epidemiology of yellow fevers in Latin America and South America. South America is classified as an endemic sector of yellow fever at the moment [19]. In Venezuela, yellow fever was presented in three wild areas: San Camilo in the Tachira State, South of the Lake in the Zulia, and Guayana [20]. In 2003, Velero noted that, according to the recording of the Health Ministry and Social Development, corresponding to the weekly epidemiological report of the year 2003, 318 yellow fever cases had been examined, of which 31 were confirmed, with a mortality rate of 58.0% [20]. Velero noted that before the appearance of this eruption, an epizooty was reported in monkeys, with a high mortality, in November of 2002 in the Semprum municipality of the Zulia State, persistent until September of 2003, with extension to the state of Tachira [20]. The high population mobilization, the remote sectors difficult to access, the high native population concentration and border conflict was proposed as the possible reasons of the re-urgence [20]. In Brazil, yellow fever is frequently associated with high severity and high mortality rates in the Amazon region [21]. During the rainy seasons of 1998 and 1999, 23 (eight deaths) and 34 (eight deaths) human cases of yellow fever were retrieved, respectively, in the different geographic sectors of the state of Para [21]. Vasconcelos et al. noted that the patients were one to 46 years old. Insects major and captured products were isolated from 4 and 11 tensions of yellow fevers, respectively, from *Haemagogus janthinomys* mosquitoes [21]. They put forth a hypothesis that yellow fever virus remained in a sector after an eruption by vertical transmission among the mosquitoes of *Haemagogus* [21]. Mondet said that the endemic sector for the yellow fever was localized to Brazil in the Amazon pool; here the cases were dispersed and were generally limited in number; nevertheless, there was also the apparition of endemic homes in this sector from which the cases were less rare, although the event remained irregular [22]. Mondet also said that the sector epidemic was mostly situated outside the Amazon pool, to the east and north and particularly to the south and the epidemics, which were all sylvatic, follow a circular pattern (in the forest sector) or a linear pattern (in the forests galleries of the savannah sector) [22]. Mondet noted that the ecological modifications that currently took place in the Amazon pool was an endemic reservoir of the virus and would inevitably facilitate an increase in the contact between the humans and the vectors [22]. Mondet concluded that while the harbor populations of more and more urban sectors of *Aedes aegypti* were at risk, it was particularly important to try to prevent contact with the human populations living in the apparition zones and the epidemic sectors, and thus prevent the arrival of the virus in the city through the humans with viremia [22].

In contrast to Asia, and the infection of dengue, the yellow fever is endemic in South America. To divide it, the mosquito vector is widely studied. Recently, Massad et al. executed an interesting study while supposing that, as a similar vector caused the two infections, all of the quantities related to the mosquito, estimated from the initial phase of dengue epidemic, could be applied to the dynamics of fever yellow, and it was shown that yellow fever was, on average, 43% less prevalent than dengue [23]. Massad et al. proposed that this difference was because of the longer viremia of dengue and the shorter incubation period [23].

E. Europe

Similar to North America, yellow fever has been eradicated in Europe for many years. However, the possible reemergence due to globalization has also been mentioned.

Vector and Transmission

Yellow fever is a viral, tropical and important illness. The infection is an illness of arbovirus [24], transmitted by *Aedes aegypti,* a mosquito that feeds inside. Historically, the test of the hypothesis of the mosquito was delayed on account of two aspects of the illness: patients are viremic only during the first several days of the clinical illness, and the majority of the mosquitoes require about two weeks for viral incubation before becoming contagious [19]. There are some recent interesting reports on the vector of yellow fever. Miller et al. reported the epidemic yellow fever caused by a vector of incompetent mosquitoes in 1989 [25]. According to this study, 27% of the experimental mosquitoes that arrived at the yellow fever epidemic area were infected, and only 7% of these transmitted the virus. By contrast, 80% of an exotic susceptible strain of *Aedes aegypti* arrived with an infected status, and 43% were capable of transmitting [25]. They also showed that none of other potential vectors were assets during the epidemic and that the local *Aedes aegypti* were present in huge numbers [25]. They concluded that an incompetent mosquito vector would be able to initiate maintain the spread of the virus with a resulting epidemic in the presence of a high density of population [25]. Tabachnick et al. carried out another study on the oral infection of *Aedes aegypti* with yellow fever virus in 1985 [26]. In this study, 28 populations that represented a world distribution of *Aedes aegypti* were tested for their ability to orally become infected with yellow fever virus [26]. According to this study, the rates of the infection suggested that populations that showed isozyme genetic relatedness also presented the similarity to oral rates of infection with yellow fever virus [26]. Tabachnick et al. concluded that their conclusions maintained the hypothesis that genetic variation existed for the oral sensitivity of yellow fever virus in the *Aedes aegypti.*

In addition to *Aedes aegypti*, there are also other vectors for the yellow fever virus. *Aedes albopictus* is another species of *Aedes* frequently mentioned as a vector for yellow fever virus [27]. In 1989, Miller et al. carried out experimental studies undertaken to identify the dynamics of yellow fever virus replica in an introduced strain (Houston) of the Asian mosquito, *Aedes albopictus,* with a hypothesis that this species was an efficient vector of yellow fever virus [28]. They concluded that the introduced strain of *Aedes albopictus* was a vector competent for yellow fever virus and could serve as vector between the wild cycle of the fever and the urban cycle in other ecosystems of the new world [28]. The vector and the possible cycles of the yellow fever infection [29] are presented in Table 1.

Table 1. Three possible cycles for yellow fever infection

Cycle	Vector	Description
Jungle (sylvatic) cycle	*Aedes* spp. (Africa), *Haemagogus* spp. (South America)	The mosquito transmits the virus to the wild non-human primates (or probably a human incidental host), and then it is transmitted to another mosquito. This cycle is limited to the humid tropical forests, and the human hosts are usually male forest workers [29].
Urban cycle	*Aedes* spp.	The mosquito transmits the virus to a human host, and then it is transmitted to another mosquito [29].
Intermediate cycle	Aedes spp.,* *Haemagogus* spp. (South America)	The mosquito transmits the virus to wild non-human primates and human hosts, and then it is transmitted to another mosquito [29]. The mosquitoes of semidomestics that live within and at the exterior of towns are the primary vectors [29]. This cycle can use a bridge between the jungle and urban sectors, spreading to the urban centers [29].

Wiwanitkit V, 2005.
* Domestic mosquito, especially *Aedes aegypti.*

In addition to vector transmission, other ways of spreading yellow fever are also mentioned. Some pregnant women can also be susceptible to yellow fever, and if they experience the illness, vertical spreading of the yellow fever virus to their babies can be expected. The intrapartum infection of yellow fever is an interesting tropical infection of the intrapartum period. Nevertheless, there is no report on the effect of intrapartum infection of yellow fever to pregnancy outcome. However, there are some investigations on the effect of yellow fever vaccination during pregnancy. In 1993, Tsai et al. carried out an interesting study in Trinidad to determine if vaccines of yellow of fever administered during pregnancy caused fetal infection during unrecognized pregnancy, in a massive campaign [30]. According to this study, maternal and cord or infant blood were tested for IgM and neutralizing antibodies to yellow fever virus, and it was found that one in 41 children had IgM and elevated neutralizing antibodies to the virus, indicating congenital infection [30]. In this study, the child, the first case report of the yellow fever infection after the immunization during pregnancy was delivered after a simple full-term pregnancy and appeared normal [30]. In conclusion, Tsai et al. noted that the frequency of the fetal infection and adverse events after such exposure would not be measureable; nevertheless, the neurotropism of virus for the development of the nervous system and the documented possibility of infection transplacentally underlined the admonition that yellow fever vaccination during pregnancy should be avoided [30]. According to the recommendations of the Advisory Committee on Immunization Practices (ACIP), 2002 [31], yellow fever vaccine during pregnancy should be considered only with special precautions.

Genetic and Molecular Biology of Yellow Fever

As previously mentioned, genetics has a significant effect on yellow fever transmission. This is one of the intrinsic factors and mechanisms underlying the capacity of vectors to transmit pathogenic agents [32]. The polymorphism in the sensitivity of expression to the oral infection was shown to vary among different geographic samples of mosquitoes [32]. It is mentioned that the intraspecific variations in vector competence were checked by one or more genes and expressed in the variable proportions in a mosquito population [32]. At this moment, the knowledge of the role of the vector in the spreading of the yellow fever virus is of interest [33]. In 2004, Vasconcelos et al. executed an analysis of 79 yellow fever virus isolates collected from 1935 to 2001 in Brazil [33]. They found that all isolates showed a single genotype (South America I) circulating in the country, with the exception of a single strain of Rondonia that represented the South America II genotype [33]. In this study, this analysis of phylogenetics indicated that the circulation of viruses vary by large geographic sectors and suggested that the migration of infected people could be an important mechanism of virus dispersion [33]. Tolou et al. noted that this study of viral genome also allowed the improvement of diagnostic techniques, the identification of factors influencing virulence, and the improvement of understanding of viral mutations [34]. The comparison of the RNA sequences of viruses among the different geographic regions showed the existence of several stable genotypes, designated as topotypes, and these topotypes nevertheless must be matched to different viral activity to allow better supervision of the epidemiology of the disease [34]. Pisano et al. recently retrieved an interesting study in West Africa [35]. In this study, three virus strains of yellow fever were isolated in 1982 in the Ivory Coast, one of a human case and two of *Aedes luteocephalus*, during and subsequent to an epidemic. Then, the genome sequence of the human strain was determined and was compared to that of Asibi strains of yellow fever [35]. The results showed the homogenity of virus strains circulating in the hosts and the different vectors in a geographically limited region and validated the concept of topotype in the almost viral types [35].

The effect of genetic polymorphism on the yellow fever vaccine also was mentioned. Bonnevie-Nielsen et al. studied 2',5'-oligoadenylate synthetase (2',5'A) activity in blood mononuclear cells (peripheral blood lymphocytes [PBLs]) from insulin-dependent diabetes mellitus (IDDM) and the checked controls [36]. They found that there was no relation between basal or stimulated 2',5'A activity and the age, the sex, the length of IDDM, the age at first of IDDM, metabolism markers, or the gene polymorphism of HLA-DQ beta-chain. Nevertheless, there was a direct relation between 2',5'A activity and latent viral infections associated with the presence of double-stranded RNA and with cellular interferons (IFNs) formed in answer to viral infections [36]. They proposed also that analysis of the activity of 2',5'A was a sensitive measure of the activation of the system of IFN and the level of latent infectivity [36]. Monath and Barrett said that the role of specific genes and molecular determinants of neurotropism and viscerotropism had been only partly defined [37]. Recently, Wang et al. examined and compared the molecular plans of three efforts to study the wild-type yellow fever viruses isolated from Senegal, called French virus of viscerotropic Rendu and Dak1279, respectively [38]. According to this study, they proposed that at least two clear genotypes of wide-type viruses had been present in Senegal. They noted that since the virus of Rendu was cut off from a fatal case of yellow fever infection, it would indicate that the vaccine-specific epitope on E protein did not associate with the extenuation of the viscerotropism of the wide-type virus [38].

Pathophysiology and Clinical Manifestation

A. Pathophysiology of Yellow Fever

The pathophysiology of yellow fever in humans is to a large extent unknown. The degree of the severity of yellow fever illness is connected with different factors related to the virus and to the receiver. With respect to the pathophysiology of the yellow fever, the virulence of the agent, yellow fever virus, is an important factor. There are some studies on the yellow fever virus virulence factors. The availability of contagious clones and a small animal (hamster) model should permit virulence factor dissemination that then can be tested in the most difficult model of the monkey [37]. Recently, Nickells and Chambers utilized a molecular clone of mouse-neuroadapted yellow fever virus17D (SPYF-MN) to identify critical determinants of neuroinvasiveness in a mouse model [39]. They found that the 3' UTR could affect the neuroinvasiveness of the SPYF virus in the mouse model [39].

In addition to agent factor, the answer or response of the host is another important factor in the pathogenesis of yellow fever. Monath and Barrett said that the role of dysregulation of cytokine and injury to the endothelium in yellow fever could be clarified as access to patients and of patients to more sophisticated medical care improves [37]. In 2004, ter Meulen et al. carried out a study to determine the contribution of provocative mediators to the pathogenesis of yellow fever [40]. In this study, the levels in the serum of various cytokines and chemokines were measured in seven patients with fatal yellow fever, 11 patients with nonfatal hemorrhage, and 18 patients with the nonfatal nonhemorrhagic form [40]. They found that the levels of interleukin (IL)-6, a protein of chemoattractant of monocytes, interferon-inducible protein, tumor necrosis factor-alpha, and IL-1 antagonist were all statistically significantly higher in the patients with fatality than in those without fatality [40]. ter Meulen et al. noted that these conclusions had implications for the comprehension of the pathophysiology and therapeutic strategies [40].

In humans, yellow fever virus replicates in Kupffer cells and in hepatocytes in the liver [40]. Xiao et al. carried out an experimental study in the animal model to study the pathology of the liver [41]. In this study, the liver showed full necrosis spots on day three after the infection, was followed by steatosis and focal confluent of necrosis and regeneration hepatocyte began on day eight, which was accompanied by decreasing steatosis [41]. The spleen initially exhibited hyperplasia of the lymphoid part, followed by lymphoid exhaustion and enlarged phagocytosis by macrophages of the spleen [41]. The focal acinar and full pancreatic necrosis, suprarenal, and cortical spotty necrosis were transitorily seen between days five and seven [41]. Xiao et al. said that TUNEL analysis showed a dynamic change of necrapoptosis of hepatocytes, corresponding to the activity and the severity of the illness [41]. Marianneau et al. noted that while the viral fever typically induced only limited the foci of necrosis in the liver, the yellow fever virus infection is characterized devastating wounds [42]. They noted that yellow fever virus grew in an exponential way at high titers and induced cytopathic changes at only 72 hours after the infection in the human hepatoma cell line [42]. Marianneau et al. said that the role of the immune response to the infection, especially cellular immunity, was characterized poorly, and the suggestion that immune clearance might aggravate the condition of the host during the period of drunkenness should be further evaluated in appropriate animal models [43].

B. Clinical Manifestations of Yellow Fever

Yellow fever is an arthropod-borne illness with symptoms that range from mild fever with acute hepatonephritis to hemorrhages and fatality [29, 43]. With regard to the infection, the classical description is a period of incubation of three to six days without prodromal symptoms [29]. The symptomatic flu-like illness then develops. The period of the infection is about three to four days [29]. Typically, the symptoms begin with fever, violent headache, discomfort, colds, anorexia, nausea, vomiting and myalgia at the lumbosacral region [29]. Fortunately, most cases will return to a phase of remission and abortive phase within one to two days [29]. About 15% of infected cases develop a period of increasing systemic symptoms, generally presenting with several complications including an episode of hemorrhage (generally recovering in five days), liver failure and renal failure and subsequent death [29]. It is noted that there is an interval between the end of the viremia and the appearance of the antibodies associated with the exacerbation of clinical symptoms, including bleeding of the mucous membranes. Digoutte noted that the rate of mortality was high for the fever with haemorrhagic episode and hepatitis, reaching 36% [45]. Digoutte also noted that the virulence of the yellow fever virus, as well as the mortality, in its wild cycle and the intermediate cycle, was greater than the urban cycle [45]. Digoutte noted that since the human is the only vertebrate host implied in the circulation of the virus in urban yellow fever, and the vector is generally *Aedes aegypti*, the domestic mosquito would be able to maintain a selective pressure, enlarging the spreading of a virus capable of producing high viremia in the human. Therefore, manifestations were more serious [45]. The clinical diagnostic evidence of yellow fever is a fever with hemorrhage and hepatitis similar to other hemorrhagic fevers such as the fever caused by Rift Valley virus [45].

Diagnosis of Yellow Fever

There have been many current advances in the diagnosis of yellow fever. Nevertheless, the basic principles in medicine—good history taking and the physical examination—are necessary. Since yellow fever can be an easily forgotten disease, awareness of this medically neglected disease is necessary [46]. The differential diagnosis of hemorrhagic fever after a history of visiting an endemic sector must include yellow fever. Microbiologically, the yellow fever virus is present in the blood of the patient during the acute phase of disease [47]. An alternate approach is the direct detection of antigen of yellow fever virus in the serum by means of ELISA [47]. At this moment, ELISA of IgM, the inhibition of ELISA and complement fixing (CF) are the tests widely used for the laboratory investigation of confirmation of yellow fever. There are some recent reports on the evaluation of these diagnostic tests. For example, Vazquez et al. recently executed a comparative study on the IgM antibody capture ELISA (MAC-ELISA) and ELISA inhibition methods, which were first developed against the dengue virus with later modifications to detect antibodies against the yellow fever virus [48]. In this study, the cross reaction was evaluated by the tests, and a high specificity to the antibodies of IgM against the yellow fever, when all of the samples of the vaccinated individuals were negative by the MAC-ELISA using the antigen of dengue, could be detected [48]. Vazquez et al. concluded that the MAC-ELISA and the inhibition methods of ELISA for the yellow fever virus could be useful for the diagnosis, supervision and vaccine evaluation of yellow fever [48]. Quantifation of yellow fever viruses is executed routinely by the virus culture to contain the samples using susceptible cells [49]. The calculation of the veneer resultant furnishes a boundary for the number of contagious particles present in the sample. In fact, the virus isolation and identification furnish a potential diagnosis method at first, but the available technics are slow and demand equipment and specialized personnel [47]. This assay usually takes five days before the results are obtained and must be executed under L2 or L3 laboratory conditions, depending on the yellow fever virus strain [49].

For the clinical diagnosis of yellow fever infection, approaches based on cell culture take too long and have limited practical relevance [49]. Regarding the molecular diagnosis of yellow fever, there have been several attempts to developed new molecular-based tests to cope with the problem of cell culture. However, most of the molecular diagnostic tools are considered expensive and not correct for the endemic sectors, which are usually poor and disadvantaged. Bae et al. noted that due to considerable sensitivity, PCR had become a promising method for virus detection. Nevertheless, while PCR could detect specific nucleic acids of viruses, it did not allow a conclusion to be drawn in regards to the potential contagiousness of the detected virus [49]. However, for diagnostic goals, a quick, virus-specific and sensitive PCR is preferable [49]. Bae et al. executed a comparative study of two independent yellow fever PCR assays in real time versus a traditional one [49]. According to this study, a significant correlation between the number of genome determined by PCR in real time and the number that corresponds to veneer in the samples was found [49]. Mendez et al. recently developed a molecular method for the diagnosis of yellow fever virus infection based on inverse transcription (RT) followed by PCR development [50]. According to the proposed method, sera were extracted with TRIZOL-LS to isolate viral RNA for further RT treatment and the PCR reaction included two primer sets designed specifically for yellow fever virus: sense primers, JM2104 (5'-CGTTGGGAGAGGAGATTC-3) and JM2249 (5'-TTCTTCACTTCGGTTGGG-3'), and antisense ones, JM2673 (5'-TCATCTGCCCTGCTTC TC-3) and JM2751 (5'-CCTCTCTGGTAAACATTCT-3) [50]. In this study, a technique to show the yellow fever virus in fabric samples was used in brains of infected mice treated with a plug of lysis before RNA extraction, and reactions of PCR were evaluated in the freezes of agarose where the single bands of the foreseen size for every pair of primers (569 bp and 502 bp) were observed [50]. Mendez et al. concluded that the RT-PCR method allowed a quick and specific demonstration of the presence of yellow fever virus [50]. Moreover, Deubel et al. reported that RT-half-nested PCR could be better used for clinical specimens for a quick and specific diagnosis, and with biopsy equipment for the retrospective studies [51].

About the histological examination, proteins of yellow fevers in the formalin-fixed and liver biopsy sunk in paraffin could be detected by the procedures of immunohistochemical test [51]. Nevertheless, the histological examination demanded invasive procedure, liver biopsy, for the collection of specimen. Therefore, it is not routine for usage.

Pathology and Complications

A. Pathology

Several pathological complications in yellow fever have been documented. The main modification is in the hematological system and hepatobiliary system, as mentioned previously. The destruction of the platelets, relating to immunopathology, is proposed. Gear said that the circulation of many infective agents—viruses—might initiate a cascade of coagulation, the formation of fibrin and their deposition in the finest blood vessels, and in the aggregate and the tangle of the platelets that have resulted as marked thrombocytopenia and bleeding [52]. Meshing noted that this bloody tendency was greatly aggravated when the infection implied specifically the cells of the parenchymal region of the liver; such a condition had as a result the faulty formation of coagulation factors such as prothrombin [52]. With regard to pathology of the liver, the predilection for cells of the midzone region of the liver lobe is noted. Some microscopic findings on the histopathology of the liver in yellow fever were previously mentioned. The role of dendritic cells in the early phase of yellow fever infection deserves attention. Vieira et al. recently studied the histopathology of the human liver in yellow fever with special diagnostic emphasis on the Councilman body [53]. In this study, liver specimens from 10 cases of yellow fever were studied by light and four by electron microscopy to revise the morphological aspects of the illness concerning the diagnosis, with the special emphasis in acidophilic bodies (AB) and in the possible presence of the virus inside infected cells [53]. According to this study, the typical modification was a necrosis of hepatocellular of AB with a preferential distribution of midzonal region [53]. The pigment of Ceroid was abundant, its quantity was proportional to degree of the damage of the liver cells, and it was found in the hepatocytes and altered Kupffer cells in the most damaged areas [53]. The provocative infiltrates were scarce, not only in tracts but also inside the lobes. The electron microscopy revealed that viral particles were found in neither cells of the liver nor in AB [53]. Vieira et al. noted that the AB, appearing as round or elliptical cytoplasmic masses, surrounded a visible cell membrane and were densely packed with organelles, fat vacuoles and residual bodies, differing from AB in other liver afflictions by the presence of vacuoles and ceroid fat pigment [53].

B. Complications

Many complications of yellow fever are documented in medicine. Renal failure, coagulopathy, the vascular instability and bleeding are examples of complications. Nevertheless, the two major common complications of yellow fever are the episodes of hemorrhage and hepatitis. The complications of hemorrhagic episodes have the fundamental mechanisms as previously mentioned. Some bleeding is fatal [54] (such as severe gastrointestinal hemorrhage). Regarding hepatitis, yellow fever is an important virus that causes hepatitis since the liver is the primary organ of the objective [55]. The clinically open dysfunction of hepatocytes is rare in this viral infection [55]. The biochemical disturbance of liver functions can be seen: rising levels of AST and ALT are frequent events and indicate liver damage [55]. The morphological changes of the liver include varying degrees of liver necrosis with a shortage of provocative activities [55]. It should be noted that necrosis at the midzonal region is rarely observed in the human liver, less so in the patients with yellow fever [56]. Nevertheless, chronic sequelae, such as the cirrhosis or hepatocellular cancer, are not found [55].

With respect to shock in severe yellow fever, the phenomenon of antibody-dependent acquaintance reaction, called “FAÇADE,” is believed to be a similar factor, contributing to dengue shock syndrome. In 1986, Barrett and Gould reported for the first time that the virus' virulence increased in mice due to utilizing monoclonal antibodies (MAbs) prepared against yellow fever virus [57]. They noted that FAÇADE was both dose-dependent of antibody and was antibody- and strain-specific [57]. In its study, a total of 12 yellow fever viruses and 11 MAbs were examined, and of these only three yellow fever viruses (FNV, Asibi and B11) could be enlarged in the live subject by only two MAbs (427 and 126) [57]. Barrett and Gould concluded that a combination of virus and antibody is required for the FAÇADE to take place. Besides, it should be noted that the necrosis of midzonal region in the liver can be a result of the shock induced by yellow fever [56].

With regard to the liver changes after the yellow fever infection in cases of death, Liu and Faucet carried out an animal model study on the effects of yellow fever [58]. In this study, marked viremia was discerned in postinoculation days (PID) 2 through 5, and the fever was first observed in PID 4 [58]. In PID 5, the volumes of blood and plasma and circulatory K + values increased, while the volume of RBC, PCV, and the concentration of the cholesterol of the plasma diminished [58]. Besides, total lipids (mainly triglycerides) accumulated in the liver of inoculated macaques; the modifications in the water in the liver content, of electrolytes, and of trace metals were observed [58]. Liu and Faucet noted that certain parts of the central nervous system (CNS), skeletal muscle, skin, heart, diaphragm, and renal bark were affected, with changes noted in the water, electrolytes, trace metals, and concentrations of lipid [58]. Liu and Faucet concluded that these changes of the weaving indicated that cell metabolism was altered and that the mechanisms of the cell membrane transportation of certain weavings were modified by yellow fever virus as the process of illness caused by the virus [58]. They proposed that the yellow fever-induced intracellular dehydration of the medulla oblongata in the subsequent phase of the illness might depress the respiratory and cardiovascular centers, thus contributing to death [58]. To confirm this hypothesis, de Brito et al. reported a study by immunohistochemical technique in the yellow fever antigen in the liver, the kidney and the heart in three fatal cases of yellow fever [59]. They noted that antigens were present in the cytoplasm of hepatocytes, of Councilman bodies and of Kupffer cells, and yellow fever antigens were also discerned in the renal tubular epithelium and in fibers of myocardium [59]. These conclusions suggest that viral replication occurs in places other than the liver [59].

Treatment

Treatment of yellow fever should be based on the severity of the infection. The concept of treatment is similar to other infections: getting rid of the pathogen or control of the infection and supportive or symptomatic treatment. In yellow fever, a specific antiviral drug for yellow fever virus is not available at present. There are some recent reports on the possible antiviral drugs for yellow fever virus infection. Sbrana et al. suggested that ribavirin might be cost-effective in the early processing of the yellow fever, and that its mechanism of action to reduce the pathology of the liver in yellow fever infection could be similar to that observed with ribavirin in the processing of the chronic infection of hepatitis C virus [60]. Nevertheless, Tuncbilek and Schneller recently noted that 5'-nor carbocyclic ribavirin was neither active nor was there cytotoxicity to the viral host cells [61]. Ono et al. recently evaluated two sulfated galactomannans, one extracted from seeds of *Mimosa scabrella*, having a mannose in proportion to the galactose of 1:1, and another with a 1:4 proportion of seeds of *Leucaena leucocephala* [62]. They found that these sulfated galactoma were shown in vitro and in vivo to work against flaviviruses [62].

Concerning supportive treatment, correction of fluid and electrolyte disturbance should be the main consideration. Similar principles to those for treatment of dengue hemorrhagic fever, another tropical mosquito-borne viral hemorrhagic disease, can be applied.

Prevention

A. Vector Control

Prevention of yellow fever is a good method to control this viral illness. Since this illness is spread by vector-borne transmission, the control of the vector is important in primary prevention. The classical methods, such as insecticide and bed nets, are extensively used in the endemic areas. Nevertheless, the application of these methods of vector control are labor intensive, require discipline and diligence, and are hard to maintain [63]. Another new alternative for vector control has been proposed. The technology of transgenesis has been developed for the mosquito of yellow fever, *Aedes aegypti* [64]. Progress is questioned with regard to the impact on public health of genetically modified mosquitoes and the ability of transformed mosquitoes to compete and to spread beneficial genes to non-transformed populations [65]. There is also a requirement for a strategy center for this genetically-based control aimed to reduce the extension to humans of mosquito-borne illness [65]. The successful integration of DNA exon in the germline of the mosquito has been achieved with the class of transposable elements, Hermes, mariner and piggyBac [64]. Adelman et al. noted that a number of marker genes, including the cinnabar(+) gene of *Drosophila melanogaster*, and fluorescent protein genes, could be utilized to control the introduction of these elements [64]. They proposed that the availability of multiple genes of elements and markers provided a powerful assembly of instruments to investigate basic biological properties of the vector insect, as well as the means to develop novel, genetic-based strategies to control the spread of the illness [64]. In 2004, Irvin et al. examined the impact of transgenesis of *Aedes aegypti*, a mosquito that transmits yellow fever [65]. They examined the effects of the elements in survival, in longevity, in fertility, in proportion of sex, and in sterility of transformed mosquitoes, and results were compared to the non-transformed ones [65]. They found that the demographic parameters are significantly diminished in the genetically-modified relative to untransformed mosquitoes [65]. Irvin et al. proposed that reduced fitness in transgenic mosquitoes had important implications for the development and the utilization of this technology for programs of control based on the manipulative molecular modification [65].

Moreover, to obtain the effective control of the vector, the precautions regarding the vector are needed. Cordellier noted that to develop systems for prevention and to permit prediction of epidemics, the inspection of sylvatic vectors for the endemic zones of each country, and identification of the type of contact between sylvatic vectors and humans in both wild and rural biotopes was necessary [66]. Cordellier also recommended other strategies, such as a) programs of basic study to detail all topotypes of the virus, and of the viral cycles of the amplification that occur again and again in various years; b) a complete map of the foci of *Stegomyia* with an evaluation of their potential risk for epidemic (an analysis of the productivity of places, depending on their type); and c) the evaluation of the immune position of the populations of the various ecosystems of each country, taking into account the past or present strategies for vaccination [66].

B. Vaccination [67]

As opposed to another mosquito-borne viral illness, an effective vaccine for yellow fever has been developed over the years. Yellow fever 17d vaccines are very common for this disease. This vaccine is shown to be cost effective for the control of yellow fever. Tomori proposed that with a 10-year period of a phase of massive campaign for vaccination against yellow fever, integrated with successful routine immunization, Africa could bring yellow fever under control [9]. Tomori noted also that for yellow fever to be eradicated, Africa should maintain at least an annual 80% rate of vaccinated children under the age of one year, and maintain a diligent system of surveillance for the illness with a sensitive program for the control of the illness [9]. Tomori also said that this could be achieved with an economic annual expense of less than US$1.00 per person [9].

Generally, yellow fever vaccine is a live viral vaccine. The recommended dosage is 0.5 ml subcutaneously. It is recommended as an inclusion in routine immunization at nine months of age in the endemic areas [68]. The international regulations of health demand a booster at 10-year intervals [68]. It is noted that this vaccine should not be given before six months of age, and the physician must avoid vaccine administration during pregnancy [68]. A certificate of vaccination is now demanded for international travel, and only for a limited number of persons [68]. Many countries demand an international vaccination validation certificate from travelers, including those in transit, arriving from infected sectors or from countries with the infected sectors [68]. Some countries demand a certificate of all travelers, even from arrivals from countries where there is no risk for yellow fever [68]. Van Laethem said that the yellow fever vaccine was the single obligatory vaccine for certain African or South American countries [69]. In many Asian countries, the vaccination is strongly advised for tourists outside the urban sectors of endemic countries if these countries have not officially documented the disease and do not demand any proof of vaccination upon entry [3,68]. On the other hand, the vaccination is also recommended before traveling to the endemic countries [3]. This vaccination remains important in travel medicine [70]. The indications of the WHO call for immunization against yellow fever at least 10 days before a trip to endemic sectors [70]. Nevertheless, Potasman et al. found that the WHO indications for the vaccination were not frequently followed [71]. They noted that an initiative to explain to the public the importance of vaccination before a trip to endemic sectors should be undertaken [71].

As previously mentioned, the vaccination is recommended only with special precautions in pregnancy. The risk of exposure to the disease must be weighed against the potential risk of the vaccine during pregnancy [68]. The vaccine is also contraindicated in immune-compromised patients and in individuals allergic to eggs [68]. Vaccination of individuals with symptomatic HIV infection is controversial. In 2004, Kemper et al. noted that HIV-infected patients must be more conscious of the necessity of medical counsel before a trip [72]. Receiver et al. documented that 17D was effective and safe in two humans infected with immunodeficiency virus without immunosuppression; one traveled to Kenya and the other traveled to Senegal [73]. Moss et al. said that the risk of serious complications from the vaccine in HIV-infected persons had not been determined [74]. In 2004, Tattevin et al. concluded that vaccine was safe and effective in HIV-infected patients [75].

Furthermore, Leder et al. noted that vaccination of elderly persons must done under special precautions since increased toxic effects following yellow fever vaccination in elderly recipients had been found [76].

Regarding unfavorable events following yellow fever vaccination, very rare cases of serious unfavorable events, including death, were recently documented. Chan et al. reported that a rapidly progressive disease with fatality could follow the administration of the 17D204 vaccine [77]. In 2001, Martin et al. documented three patients who disease within days after vaccination [78]. The clinical presentations were characterized by fever, myalgia, headache, and confusion, followed by severe multisystemic disorders [78]. These three patients died, and varying vaccine-related variants of yellow fever viruses were found in the plasma and cerebrospinal fluid of a vaccinee [78]. Furthermore, the convalescent samples of serum of two vaccines showed responses to the antibody of at least 1:10240 and assay of fabric immunohistochemistry of liver showed the yellow fever antigen in the Kuppfer cells [78]. Martin et al. concluded that the clinical characteristics, the temporal association with the vaccination, the virus restoration of related vaccine, the antibody responses, and the assay of immunohistochemistry suggested a possible causal relationship between the disease and the vaccination [78]. Martin et al. also noted that advanced age could be a risk factor for the disease temporally associated with yellow fever vaccination [79]. In 2004, Lawrence et al. noted that the unfavorable events following vaccination had raised the concern regarding vaccine safety, particularly among the oldest vaccines [78]. They examined the age-related reporting rates of adverse events following YF vaccination reported to the Australian Adverse Drug Reactions Advisory Committee for the period 1993 to 2002 and found that the highest reported rates occurred among the oldest vaccines [78]. Although there are reports on the unfavorable effects of vaccination, the risk to unimmunized individuals and to those traveling to sectors known for transmission is much greater than the risk for having a vaccine-related unfavorable event [68].

References

[1] Vasconcelos PF. Yellow Fever. *Rev. Soc. Bras. Med. Trop.* 36, 275-93 (2003)

[2] Monath TP. Yellow fever: an update. *Lancet. Infect. Dis.* 1, 11-20 (2001)

[3] Wiwanitkit V. Amazing Thailand Year 1998-1999 Tourist's health concepts. *Chula. Med. J.* 42, 975-984 (1998)

[4] Grendel D. Vaccinations for the travellers. *Rev. Prat.* 54, 519-25 (2004)

[5] Hatz C. Medical travel counseling and vaccinations. *Schweiz. Rundsch. Med. Prax.* 89, 868-77 (2000)

[6] Gubler DJ. The changing epidemiology of yellow fever and dengue, 1900 to 2003: full circle? *Comp. Immunol. Microbiol. Infect. Dis.* 27, 319-30 (2004)

[7] Barrett AD, Monath TP. Epidemiology and ecology of yellow fever virus. *Adv. Virus. Res.* 61, 291-315 (2003)

[8] Mutebi JP, Barrett AD. The epidemiology of yellow fever in Africa. *Microbes. Infect.* 4, 1459-68 (2002)

[9] Tomori O. Yellow fever in Africa: public health impact and prospects for control in the 21st century. *Biomedica.* 22, 178-210 (2002)

[10] Sang RC, Dunster LM. The growing threat of arbovirus transmission and outbreaks in Kenya: a review. *East. Afr. Med. J.* 78, 655-61 (2001)

[11] Onyango CO, Grobbelaar AA, Gibson GV, Sang RC, Sow A, Swaneopel R, Burt FJ.Yellow fever outbreak, southern Sudan, 2003. *Emerg. Infect. Dis.* 10, 1668-70 (2004)

[12] Pandit CG. India and the yellow fever problem. *Indian. J. Med. Res.* 5,1523-47 (1971)

[13] Kumar S. Yellow fever threat in India. *Lancet.* 2001 Apr 28;357(9265):1346. (2001)

[14] Banerjee K. Emerging viral infections with special reference to India. *Indian. J. Med. Res.* 103, 177-200 (1996)

[15] Downs WG. The known and the unknown in yellow fever ecology and epidemiology. *Ecol. Dis.* 1, 103-10 (1982)

[16] Tomori O. Yellow fever: the recurring plague. *Crit. Rev. Clin. Lab. Sci.* 41, 391-427 (2004)

[17] Newsom EY. South Carolina's last yellow fever epidemic: Manning Simons at Port Royal, 1877. *JSC. Med. Assoc.* 91, 311-3 (1995)

[18] Monath TP. Facing up to re-emergence of urban yellow fever. *Lancet.* 353, 1541 (1999)

[19] Bryan CS, Moss SW, Kahn RJ. Yellow fever in the Americas. *Infect. Dis. Clin. North. Am.* 18, 275-92 (2004)

[20] Valero N. Yellow fever in Venezuela. *Invest. Clin.* 44, 269-71 (2003)

[21] Vasconcelos PF, Rosa AP, Rodrigues SG, Rosa ES, Monteiro HA, Cruz AC, Barros VL, Souza MR, Rosa JF. Yellow fever in Para State, Amazon region of Brazil, 1998-1999: entomologic and epidemiologic findings. *Emerg. Infect. Dis.* 7(3 Suppl), 565-9 (2001)

[22] Mondet B. Yellow fever epidemiology in Brazil. *Bull. Soc. Pathol. Exot.* 94, 260-7 (2001)

[23] Massad E, Burattini MN, Coutinho FA, Lopez LF. Dengue and the risk of urban yellow fever reintroduction in Sao Paulo State, Brazil. *Rev. Saude. Publica.* 37, 477 - 84 (2003)

[24] Kurane I. Yellow fever virus. *Nippon. Rinsho.* 61 Suppl 3, 494-6 (2003)

[25] Miller BR, Monath TP, Tabachnick WJ, Ezike VI. Epidemic yellow fever caused by an incompetent mosquito vector. *Trop. Med. Parasitol.* 40, 396-9 (1989)

[26] Tabachnick WJ, Wallis GP, Aitken TH, Miller BR, Amato GD, Lorenz L, Powell JR, Beaty BJ. Oral infection of Aedes aegypti with yellow fever virus: geographic variation and genetic considerations. *Am. J. Trop. Med. Hyg.* 34, 1219-24 (1985)

[27] Johnson BW, Chambers TV, Crabtree MB, Filippis AM, Vilarinhos PT, Resende MC, Macoris Mde L, Miller BR. Vector competence of Brazilian Aedes aegypti and Ae. albopictus for a Brazilian yellow fever virus isolate. *Trans. R. Soc. Trop. Med. Hyg.* 96, 611-3 (2002)

[28] Miller BR, Mitchell CJ, Ballinger ME. Replication, tissue tropisms and transmission of yellow fever virus in Aedes albopictus. *Trans. R. Soc. Trop. Med. Hyg.* 83, 252-5 (1989)

[29] Shoff WH. Yellow fever. Available at http://www.emedicine.com/ped/topic2463.htm

[30] Tsai TF, Paul R, Lynberg MC, Letson GW. Congenital yellow fever virus infection after immunization in pregnancy. *J. Infect. Dis.* 168, 1520-3 (1993)

[31] Cetron MS, Marfin AA, Julian KG, Gubler DJ, Sharp DJ, Barwick RS, Weld LH, Chen R, Clover RD, Deseda-Tous J, Marchessault V, Offit PA, Monath TP. Yellow fever vaccine. Recommendations of the Advisory Committee on Immunization Practices (ACIP), 2002. *MMWR. Recomm. Rep.* 51(RR-17), 1-11 (2002)

[32] Failloux AB, Vazeille-Falcoz M, Mousson L, Rodhain F. Genetic control of vectorial competence in Aedes mosquitoes. *Bull. Soc. Pathol. Exot.* 92, 266-73 (1999)

[33] Vasconcelos PF, Bryant JE, da Rosa TP, Tesh RB, Rodrigues SG, Barrett AD. Genetic divergence and dispersal of yellow fever virus, Brazil. *Emerg. Infect. Dis.* 10, 1578-84 (2004)

[34] Tolou H, Pisano MR, Durand JP. Molecular epidemiology of yellow fever. *Med. Trop. (Mars).* 58(2 Suppl), 37-41 (1998)

[35] Pisano MR, Nicoli J, Tolou H. Homogeneity of yellow fever virus strains isolated during an epidemic and a post-epidemic period in West Africa. *Virus. Genes.* 14, 225-34 (1997)

[36] Bonnevie-Nielsen V, Larsen ML, Frifelt JJ, Michelsen B, Lernmark A. Association of IDDM and attenuated response of 2',5'-oligoadenylate synthetase to yellow fever vaccine. *Diabetes.* 38, 1636-42 (1989)

[37] Monath TP, Barrett AD. Pathogenesis and pathophysiology of yellow fever. *Adv. Virus. Res.* 60, 343-95 (2003)

[38] Wang H, Jennings AD, Ryman KD, Late CM, Wang E, Ni H, Minor PD, Barrett AD. Genetic variation among strains of wild-type yellow fever virus from Senegal. *J. Gen. Virol.* 78 (Pt 6),1349-52 (1997)

[39] Nickells M, Chambers TJ. Neuroadapted yellow fever virus 17D: determinants in the envelope protein govern neuroinvasiveness for SCID mice. *J. Virol.* 77, 12232-42 (2003)

[40] ter Meulen J, Sakho M, Koulemou K, Magassouba N, Bah A, Preiser W, Daffis S, Klewitz C, Bae HG, Niedrig M, Zeller H, Heinzel-Gutenbrunner M, Koivogui L, Kaufmann A. Activation of the cytokine network and unfavorable outcome in patients with yellow fever. *J. Infect. Dis.* 190, 1821-7 (2004)

[41] Xiao SY, Zhang H, Guzman H, Tesh RB. Experimental yellow fever virus infection in the Golden hamster (Mesocricetus auratus). II. Pathology. *J. Infect. Dis.* 183, 1437-44 (2001)

[42] Marianneau P, Steffan AM, Royer C, Drouet MT, Kirn A, Deubel V. Differing infection patterns of dengue and yellow fever viruses in a human hepatoma cell line. *J. Infect. Dis.* 178, 1270-8 (1998)

[43] Marianneau P, Despres P, Deubel V. Recent knowledge on the pathogenesis of yellow fever and questions for the future. *Bull. Soc. Pathol. Exot.* 92(5 Pt 2), 432-4 (1999)

[44] Nassar Eda S, Chamelet EL, Coimbra TL, de Souza LT, Suzuki A, Ferreira IB, da Silva MV, Rocco IM, Travassos da Rosa AP. Jungle yellow fever: clinical and laboratorial studies emphasizing viremia on a human case. *Rev. Inst. Med. Trop. Sao. Paulo.* 37, 337-41 (1995)

[45] Digoutte JP. Present status of an arbovirus infection: yellow fever, its natural history of hemorrhagic fever, Rift Valley fever. *Bull. Soc. Pathol. Exot.* 92, 343-8 (1999)

[46] Monath TP. Yellow fever: a medically neglected disease. Report on a seminar. *Rev. Infect. Dis.* 9, 165-75 (1987)

[47] Monath TP, Nystrom RR. Detection of yellow fever virus in serum by enzyme immunoassay. *Am. J. Trop. Med. Hyg.* 33, 151-7 (1984)

[48] Vazquez S, Valdes O, Pupo M, Delgado I, Alvarez M, Pelegrino JL, Guzman MG. MAC-ELISA and ELISA inhibition methods for detection of antibodies after yellow fever vaccination. *J. Virol. Methods.* 110, 179-84 (2003)

[49] Bae HG, Nitsche A, Teichmann A, Biel SS, Niedrig M. Detection of yellow fever virus: a comparison of quantitative real-time PCR and plaque assay. *J. Virol. Methods.* 110, 185-91 (2003)

[50] Mendez JA, Rodriguez G, Bernal Mdel P, de Calvache D, Boshell J. Molecular detection of yellow fever virus in human sera and mice brains. *Biomedica.* 23, 232-8 (2003)

[51] Deubel V, Huerre M, Cathomas G, Drouet MT, Wuscher N, Le Guenno B, Widmer AF. Molecular detection and characterization of yellow fever virus in blood and liver specimens of a non-vaccinated fatal human case. *J. Med. Virol.* 53, 212-7 (1997)

[52] Gear JH. Hemorrhagic fevers, with special reference to recent outbreaks in southern Africa. *Rev. Infect. Dis.* 1, 571-91 (1979)

[53] Vieira WT, Gayotto LC, de Lima CP, de Brito T. Histopathology of the human liver in yellow fever with special emphasis on the diagnostic role of the Councilman body. *Histopathology.* 7, 195-208 (1983)

[54] Colebunders R, Mariage JL, Coche JC, Pirenne B, Kempinaire S, Hantson P, Van Gompel A, Niedrig M, Van Esbroeck M, Bailey R, Drosten C, Schmitz H. A Belgian traveler who acquired yellow fever in the Gambia. *Clin. Infect. Dis.* 35, e113-6 (2002)

[55] Tandon BN, Acharya SK. Viral diseases involving the liver. *Baillieres. Clin. Gastroenterol.* 1, 211-30 (1987)

[56] de la Monte SM, Arcidi JM, Moore GW, Hutchins GM. Midzonal necrosis as a pattern of hepatocellular injury after shock. *Gastroenterology.* 86, 627-31 (1984)

[57] Barrett AD, Gould EA. Antibody-mediated early death in vivo after infection with yellow fever virus. *J. Gen. Virol.* 67 (Pt 11), 2539-42 (1986)

[58] Liu CT, Griffin MJ. Changes in body fluid compartments, tissue water and electrolyte distribution, and lipid concentrations in rhesus macaques with yellow fever. *Am. J. Vet. Res.* 43, 2013-8 (1982)

[59] De Brito T, Siqueira SA, Santos RT, Nassar ES, Coimbra TL, Alves VA. Human fatal yellow fever. Immunohistochemical detection of viral antigens in the liver, kidney and heart. *Pathol. Res. Pract.* 188, 177-81 (1992)

[60] Sbrana E, Xiao SY, Guzman H, Ye M, Travassos da Rosa AP, Tesh RB. Efficacy of post-exposure treatment of yellow fever with ribavirin in a hamster model of the disease. *Am. J. Trop. Med. Hyg.* 71, 306-12 (2004)

[61] Tuncbilek M, Schneller SW. 5'-nor carbocyclic ribavirin. Nucleosides Nucleotides *Nucleic. Acids.* 22, 1995-2001 (2003)

[62] Ono L, Wollinger W, Rocco IM, Coimbra TL, Gorin PA, Sierakowski MR. In vitro and in vivo antiviral properties of sulfated galactomannans against yellow fever virus (BeH111 strain) and dengue 1 virus (Hawaii strain). *Antiviral. Res.* 60, 201-8 (2003)
[63] Guzman MG, Mune M, Kouri G. Dengue vaccine: priorities and progress. *Expert. Rev. Anti. Infect. Ther.* 2, 895-911 (2004)
[64] Adelman ZN, Jasinskiene N, James AA. Development and applications of transgenesis in the yellow fever mosquito, Aedes aegypti. *Mol. Biochem. Parasitol.* 121, 1-10 (2002)
[65] Irvin N, Hoddle MS, O'Brochta DA, Carey B, Atkinson PW. Assessing fitness costs for transgenic Aedes aegypti expressing the GFP marker and transposase genes. *Proc. Natl. Acad. Sci. USA.* 101, 891-6 (2004)
[66] Cordellier R. Yellow fever in Western Africa, 1973-1987. Observed facts--studies realized, campaign, prevention and forecast. *World. Health. Stat. Q.* 43, 52-67 (1990)
[67] Wiwanitkit V. Vaccination against mosquito borne viral infections: current status. *Iran. J. Immunol.* 4, 186 – 96 (2007)
[68] WHO. Yellow fever vaccine. Available at http://www.who.int/vaccines/en/ yellowfever.shtml
[69] Van Laethem Y. Vaccinations for the traveler. *J. Pharm. Belg.* 57,130-4. (2002)
[70] Kirkpatrick BD, Alston WK. Current immunizations for travel. *Curr. Opin. Infect. Dis.* 16, 369-74 (2003)
[71] Potasman I, Pick N, Stringer C, Zuckerman JN. Inadequate protection against yellow fever of children visiting endemic areas. *Am. J. Trop. Med. Hyg.* 65, 954-7 (2001)
[72] Kemper CA, Linett A, Kane C, Deresinski SC. Travels with HIV: the compliance and health of HIV-infected adults who travel. *Int. J. STD. AIDS.* 8, 44-9 (1997)
[73] Receveur MC, Thiebaut R, Vedy S, Malvy D, Mercie P, Bras ML. Yellow fever vaccination of human immunodeficiency virus-infected patients: report of 2 cases. *Clin. Infect. Dis.* 31, E7-8 (2000)
[74] Moss WJ, Clements CJ, Halsey NA. Immunization of children at risk of infection with human immunodeficiency virus. *Bull. World. Health. Organ.* 81, 61-70(2003)
[75] Tattevin P, Depatureaux AG, Chapplain JM, Dupont M, Souala F, Arvieux C, Poveda JD, Michelet C. Yellow fever vaccine is safe and effective in HIV-infected patients. *AIDS.* 18, 825-7 (2004)
[76] Leder K, Weller PF, Wilson ME. Travel vaccines and elderly persons: review of vaccines available in the United States. *Clin. Infect. Dis.* 33, 1553-66 (2001)
[77] Chan RC, Penney DJ, Little D, Carter IW, Roberts JA, Rawlinson WD. Hepatitis and death following vaccination with 17D-204 yellow fever vaccine. *Lancet.* 358, 121-2 (2001)
[78] Martin M, Tsai TF, Cropp B, Chang GJ, Holmes DA, Tseng J, Shieh W, Zaki SR, Al-Sanouri I, Cutrona AF, Ray G, Weld LH, Cetron MS. Fever and multisystem organ failure associated with 17D-204 yellow fever vaccination: a report of four cases. *Lancet.* 358, 98-104 (2001)
[79] Martin M, Weld LH, Tsai TF, Mootrey GT, Chen RT, Niu M, Cetron MS; GeoSentinel Yellow Fever Working Group. Advanced age a risk factor for illness temporally associated with yellow fever vaccination. *Emerg. Infect. Dis.* 7, 945-51 (2001)

[80] Lawrence GL, Burgess MA, Kass RB. Age-related risk of adverse events following yellow fever vaccination in Australia. *Commun. Dis. Intell.* 28, 244-8 (2004)

Chapter VI

West Nile Virus Infection

Introduction to West Nile Virus Infection

West Nile virus infection is a mosquito-borne infection. This infection is a new emerging viral infection. The infection of this virus is caused by a flavivirus transmitted from birds to humans by the bite of culicine mosquitoes [1]. The West Nile virus was discovered in the blood of a feverish woman of the Western province of the Nile in Uganda in 1937 [1]. The West Nile virus can cause West Nile fever in humans, in a small proportion (around one in 150), and the illness can take a course associated with severe symptoms of the central nervous system (encephalitis) and even death, especially in older patients (> 70 years) [2]. While the majority of the humans infected with West Nile virus are asymptomatic, some can develop an influenza-like illness [1]. Caution surrounding the illness remains the cornerstone of the recognition and early control of West Nile virus [1]. The birds serve as the deposit for the West Nile virus and the spreading of the virus occurs predominantly by mosquitoes [2]. Ornithophilic mosquitoes transmit the virus among the population of birds, while those species of mammals that feed off the birds can also transmit the pathogen to humans [2]. Nevertheless, mammals are considered to be dead ends that do not contribute to the extension of the epidemic of the pathogen [2]. At present, prevention and control are the only measures that help to diminish the morbidity and the mortality associated with West Nile virus infection [1]. When the number of cases is aggravated and the geographical distribution of the West Nile virus infection widens, the epidemic will continue to place a greater challenge to clinicians in the future years [1]. Guharoy et al. said that there was an urgent need for more investigation into the pathogenesis and the processing of the West Nile virus infection [1]. The western infection of the Nile virus is a zoonosis and cannot be easily eradicated. Utilizing vaccine to avoid transmission to humans is not available at present. The true mechanisms of the illness of West Nile virus infection were poorly understood and had not been the subject of modern clinical investigation [2]. Truly, West Nile virus is a small virus of single-strand RNA and a member of the antigenic complex of encephalitis virus [1]. King et al. said that a member of the neurotropic serocomplex of Japanese encephalitis infection causes the functional changes associated with the enlarged efficacy of the immune response, which subverts or avoids the immune system of the host [3]. The knowledge of West Nile virus infection is, therefore, an interesting theme for general practitioners throughout the world.

The spread of West Nile virus in North America since 1999 has raised public concern about this pathogen in Europe [2]. In contrast to the United States, where the virus has spread from New York throughout the continent to the west coast, only temporally and regionally limited outbreaks of West Nile virus infections have been observed in Europe since the 1950s [2]. The differences so far observed between the epidemics in North America and in Europe might be described by the following: Europe has had long contact with West Nile virus-rich areas in Africa, owing to migratory birds, whereas the virus was first imported into the United States in 1999 where it infected a "naïve" bird population [2]. It is possible that the strain presently spreading through the United States is highly pathogenic, whereas strains of various pathogenic potential circulate in Africa [2]. This could result in a natural immunization of the avian population through coming into contact with strains of low pathogenicity [2]. The possibility of a natural resistance in European birds is also being considered, since these animals have been in contact with the virus for long periods of time [2]. Investigations on the prevalence and incidence of West Nile virus infections in German avian populations as well as in no-way-out hosts such as humans and horses could provide information regarding the potential risk posed by West Nile virus [2].

Worldwide Epidemiology of West Nile Virus Infection

West Nile virus is a common arbovirosis in sub-Saharian Africa. It has occasionally caused epidemics or epizootics in horses in Mediterranean regions and southern Europe [4]. This disease has become an important new emerging contagious disease in many Western countries in recent years. Unlike other tropical mosquito-borne infections, the risk for introduction and spread of West Nile virus infection to the Western hemisphere is proposed due to the migration of birds. A summary on some recent reports on the epidemiology of West Nile virus infections in several regions of the world are hereby presented.

A. Asia

Although Asia is the endemic area of the Japanese encephalitis virus infection, it is not the endemic area for West Nile infection. Nevertheless, there are some recent reports of the epidemic in the area neighboring Africa. There are many reports with respect to West Nile virus in southern Asia, an important endemic area of Japanese encephalitis. The possible role of birds in the conservation of West Nile virus has been also described in India [5]. They noted that although Japanese encephalitis virus was found to dominate in the southern part of India, very few clinically open cases of human encephalitis due to West Nile virus were observed. Moreover, West Nile fever in horses has never been documented in India [5]. In 2003, Jamgaonkar et al. carried out an inspection of serology of birds in a Japanese encephalitis endemic area of the District of Kolar, State of Karnataka, India [6]. In this study,

859 birds were tested by hemagglutination inhibition for Japanese encephalitis and West Nile virus. Two (0.002%) and 178 (20.72%) were positive for the Japanese encephalitis virus and West Nile virus, respectively [6]. Jamgaonkar et al. concluded that many species of birds among terrestrial birds were infected with West Nile virus and probably played a role in the conservation of the virus in the previously-mentioned part of India [6]. In 2002, Thakare et al. carried out another study to document the frequency of West Nile virus in India [7]. During the investigation by virological method of cases of suspected viral fever carried out at the National Institute of Virology (NIV) in Pune, India, evidence of recent infection with West Nile virus was discerned in 88 cases [7].

With respect to the Middle East, an area more to the west of Asia than to Africa, there are some reports of a sudden spike in West Nile virus cases. Malkinson et al. recently proposed the introduction of West Nile virus to white Middle East emigrating storks [8]. In the study, West Nile virus was isolated in a multitude of emigrating white storks that landed in Eilat, a town in southern Israel [8]. The 13 dead persons or dying storks came into contact two days after the arrival and they were submitted to laboratory for exam; four West Nile viruses were obtained from brains [8]. Malkinson et al. said that these storks emigrated toward the south for the first time and they had not flown over Israel, so it is assumed that they had been infected with the virus at some point in their route of migration over Europe [8]. In the summer of 2000, a sharp increase in West Nile virus cases were identified in the northern and central parts of Israel, affecting 439 people, with 29 fatal cases, mainly older people [9]. According to this spike, the analysis of the succession, and phylogenetics that covers the PreM, M, and part of the genes, they revealed two lineages: one narrowly related to a 1999 Israeli bird (seagull) segment and a 1999 bird from New York (the flamenco) segment; and the other narrowly related to a 1997 Romanian mosquito segment and a 1999 Russian human brain segment [9]. Bin et al. proposed a pattern of seroprevalence of a) 86% in people that had close contact with sick geese; b) 28% in people in areas near the route of the bird migration; and c) 27% of the general population in Israel, implying the importance of geese to human spreading [9]. With respect to the outbreak in 2000, Weinberger et al. said that cases were distributed throughout the land; men and women were equally disturbed [10]. They noted that incidence per 1,000 population increased from 0.01 in the first decade of life to 0.87 in the ninth decade [10]. In this outbreak, age-specific case death rate increased with age [10]. In 1977, Meco studied antibodies against West Nile virus in 937 sera from different persons in southeast Anatolia, Turkey, and the West Nile antibodies could be detected in 41.80% [11]. In this study, Meco also noted that the positive ratio increased according to age [11]. Concerning the other parts of Asia, Southeast Asia and East Asia, no reports of the emergence of West Nile virus infection can be found.

B. Africa

Africa is the endemic area for many mosquito-borne illnesses, including the infection of West Nile virus. According to previously mentioned words, Africa is believed to be the origin of this viral infection. Malkinson and Banet knew the importance of the bird in the spreading within and beyond of Africa [12]. They said that the unique sensitivity of young domestic geese in Israel in 1997–2000 to the virus and the isolation of similar strains from the white storks of the migration in Israel and Egypt suggested that the recent infections were more pathogenic for certain species of avians and that the migrating birds played a crucial role in the geographical extension of the virus [12]. They observed that the knowledge of the routes taken by the birds that migrate between Africa and Europe, therefore, would help in selecting the locations that would be the most fruitful in attempting to isolating the virus [12]. McLean et al. they said that the West Nile virus appeared to be maintained in endemic foci in the African continent and that it was transported yearly to the temperate climates northward in Europe and southward in South Africa [13].

There have been many reports on the recent infections of West Nile virus in many tropical countries in Africa. In Sudan, there was a recent outbreak in 2002 [14]. Depoortere et al. said that there were many unique aspects of the infection of this virus in Sudan, including the occurrence of the illness only between children and the clinical domination of encephalitis, implying severe neurological sequelae [14]. In the autumn of 1997, an epidemic of West Nile fever occurred in the area of Sfax (southeast Tunisia) [15]. In this epidemic, 57 patients were hospitalized with meningitis and/or aseptic encephalitis [15]. Feki et al. found that the rate of seropositivity of the patients with West Nile virus was 23.4%, and the forecast of the implication of the central nervous system (CNS) during the fever phase of infection seemed to be poor in elderly patients [15].

Referring to the infection in horses, Guthrie et al. studied 488 young purebred horses and found that approximately 11% of yearly viral seroconversion of the West Nile virus in the coupled samples of serum collected from each animal separated by approximately 12 months could be seen [16]. They said that the infection of horses with the virus was common in South Africa, but the infection was not associated with neurological illness [16].

C. North America

The first case of domestically acquired Wile Nile virus infection was reported in the United States in 1999 in New York [1]. Historically, the West Nile fever arose in New York and to two surrounding counties of New York in the summer of 1999, when seven people, various horses and thousands of wild birds died [17-18]. Simultaneously, an epizootic outbreak between American ravens and another species of bird occurred in four states [17-18]. Marfin and Gubler said that the native transmission of the disease had never been documented in the Western hemisphere prior to this epidemic [18]. Soon it was established that the human illness and the mortality of birds were related [17]. In 2000, the epizootic widened to 12 states and to the District of Columbia, and the epidemic continued in New York City, in five counties of New Jersey, and in one county of Connecticut [18]. Since then, the West Nile virus infection has scattered quickly through the United States, with 9,306 cases confirmed and 210 deaths reported from 45 states in 2003 [1, 19]. Many of the West Nile virus endeavors during recent outbreaks showed a very high degree of homologue that totally suggests the widespread circulation of potentially epidemic efforts of West Nile virus [18]. Guharoy noted that it was yet not clear how West Nile virus was introduced in North America [1]. The high rates of the illness and the severe neurological death among humans, horses and birds in these outbreaks were also unheard-of and unexplained [18]. The caution continued in the monitoring of the infection in mosquitoes, birds, horses, small mammals, bats and humans, and has shown its extension to various states [17, 19-20].

In additional to the United States, the infection is also documented to newly arise as an emerging contagious illness in Canada [21]. In July to September, 2002, an outbreak of West Nile virus caused a high number of deaths in Canada [22]. During the 2002 outbreak, Condotta et al. compared combined and individual samples of two species of the mosquitoes (*Culex pipiens* and *Culex restuans*) gathered from three regions by the Unit of the Health in Ontario, Canada [23]. According to this study, significantly more *restuans* were infected with West Nile virus compared to *pipiens* [23]. With regard to the human infection in Canada, in 2003, in seven patients with West Nile virus, the neurological manifestations were recently identified by the consulting services of the neurology department at the hospital in Calgary, Alberta [24].

D. South America

Although it is the endemic area for many mosquito-borne illnesses, South America is not the endemic area of the West Nile virus infection. No report of West Nile virus infections in South America have been discerned.

E. Europe

Similar to North America, West Nile virus infection has become a new emerging disease in Europe. It has been described occasionally in southern Europe and in some Mediterranean countries [25]. Hubalek and Halouzka said that West Nile infection cases and the sporadic outbreaks caused illness in humans and horse in Europe (western Russia, Mediterranean and southern Europe in 1962–64, Belarus and Ukraine in the 1970s and 1980s, Romania in 1996–97, the Czech Republic in 1997, and Italy in 1998) [26]. They said that various environmental factors, including human activities that enlarged the vector mosquito's population density (heavy rains followed by floods, irrigation, higher than usual temperature, or the formation of niches of ecology that permit a mass rise of mosquitoes) would be able to increase the incidence of the West Nile fever [26]. Durand et al. said that West Nile virus clinical aspects seem to change with an increase of the central neurological participation and a higher mortality, especially among people older than 50 years, since 1994 [25]. In France, the recent infections have been discerned in birds controlled by sentry in 2001 and 2002 [27]. As a consequence of an epizootic equine in Camargue in 2000, the French medical authorities documented an inspection of the circulation of West Nile virus in the south of France [25]. During 2003, this efficient action resulted in the identification of six human cases in a previously virus-free area in France and along the Mediterranean coast, but not in Camargue [25].

In Russia, there are also some reports in the epidemiology of West Nile virus infection. Lvov et al. said that extensive outbreaks of the epidemic of the West Nile fever with an exceptionally high mortality appeared in the last few years in Russia, especially in the southern part [28]. The West Nile virus was discovered in three species of complete birds in the summer–autumn, 2002, in the South of Western Siberia [29]. The nucleotide sequence of the 300–472 fragment of amino acid of the protein gene of the virus showed the maximum level of homologue with the WNV/LEIV-Vlg99-27889 that was taken from a patient in Volgograd in 1999 [29]. According to these reports, the importance of the migration of birds in the spread of West Nile virus in Russia can be indicated.

F. Australia

Concerning the West Nile virus infection in Australia, it is also noted as an important emerging infectious disease [30-31]. Zeller and Schuffenecker said that strains from lineage I were present in Africa and India and were responsible for the outbreaks in Europe, Australia and in the Mediterranean basin [30]. Infection of Kunjin virus, a subtype of West Nile virus, is also common in Australia [32].

Vector and Transmission

The West Nile virus is one of the arboviruses, more ubiquitous and occurring over a wide geographical range and in a wide diversity of vertebrate hosts and species of vector [13]. This disease is a viral, tropical and important illness. Transmitted by the *Culex* mosquito, this neurotropic virus affects predominantly the CNS. As previously mentioned, the migration of birds has been the important path in spreading the illnesses of this virus throughout its history. In the Western hemisphere, the infection of this virus has been diagnosed and has been mentioned in relation to migration from endemic areas in recent years. Humans, horses, birds, and vector mosquitoes are the important components in the infection. The West Nile virus is an important arthropod–borne flavivirus, generally causing a mild infection called West Nile fever in the human and horses [5]. The mosquitoes are the main vectors of West Nile virus [5]. Several species of *Culex* are found to act as vectors in different geographical regions [5]. The experimental studies had shown that *Culex tritaeniorhynchus*, *Culex vishnui*, *Culex bitaeniorhynchus* and *Culex univittatus*, *Culex pipiens fatigans* and *Aedes albopictus* would be able to act as potential vectors West Nile virus [5]. The transovarial spread of West Nile virus has been experimentally shown in *Culex* mosquitoes [5]. Aside from mosquitoes, the role of other arthropods is considered also in the conservation of West Nile virus during periods of buries-enzootic [5]. Of interest, the virus is maintained in a cycle of bird-mosquito in nature [5]. The virus is transmitted to humans by the mosquitoes that become infected by biting birds of viremic stage [4].

There are some recent interesting reports in the epidemiology of the West Nile virus infection. Recently, Peterson et al. utilized a shaping study to investigate the spreading of the infection of this virus in the United States [33]. They found that the situation with mosquitoes only did not coincide with guidelines observed in the extension, while the other with mosquitoes and migratory birds coincided, suggesting that the guidelines observed in the extension were better explained with migratory birds as agents of long distance transportation; the virus, in regions to which it was transported by migratory birds, then was transmitted enzootically to mosquitoes [33]. Brownstein et al. carried out another spatial analysis of West Nile virus for the evaluation of the risk of vector-borne introduced zoonosis [34]. They found that logistic regression analysis revealed a satellite-derived vegetation to be significantly and positively strongly associated with the presence of human cases [34].

Besides the spread owing to vectors, other means of transmitting the West Nile virus are also mentioned. In animals, Banet-Noach et al. suggested that horizontal transmission of West Nile virus could occur in commercial multitudes and might be aggravated if the cannibalism and feather-plucking of sick geese occurred [35]. New mechanisms of transmission by blood donation, organ transplant, and by the intrauterine routes have also been reported [27]. The possible spread from the mother to infant through breast milk is also mentioned [36]. Some pregnant women can also be susceptible to the virus, and if they experience the infection the vertical transmission of West Nile virus infection to their infants can be expected. The intrapartum infection of West Nile virus is interesting in obstetrics. A report that describes a case of transplacental West Nile transmission was noted in 2002 [36]. It is noted that pregnant women should take precautions to reduce the risk of West Nile virus or another infection of the arboviral group and should be tested when clinically appropriate [36]. In 2002, a woman who had West Nile encephalitis during the 27th week of her pregnancy delivered a full-term boy with chorioretinitis, the cystic destruction of the cerebral weaving, and the laboratory evidence showed the congenitally-acquired infection of West Nile virus [37-38]. Although this case demonstrated the intrauterine West Nile virus infection in a boy with congenital abnormalities, it did not show a causal relationship between the infection and any abnormalities [38]. In 2003, Alpert et al. said that intrauterine transmission of West Nile virus might have as a result a significant morbidity of ocular and neurological systems [37]. They noted that the titers for this important pathogen should be obtained when standard serology was negative in a boy with marking congenital abnormalities of the chorioretinal organ [37]. In 2004, the Central for Disease Control and Prevention (CDC) proposed provisional guidelines for the evaluation of children born to mothers infected with West Nile virus during pregnancy [38]. During 2002, the CDC investigated three cases of maternal West Nile virus infection and found that the children were born full term with normal appearance and negative laboratory tests for the infection of virus among all samples [38]. In 2002, the CDC also proposed a case of possible spreading of the virus to a boy by breastfeeding [39]. In this case, the boy was exposed to the mother's milk and was found to be infected with the West Nile virus by TaqMan molecular test [40].

With regards to the transmission via blood and blood products, transfusion-associated transmission of West Nile virus was first identified in the United States in 2002 [41]. In 2003, the agencies for the collection of blood responded by investigation of West Nile virus by utilizing nucleic acid-amplification tests (NATs) [41]. The pooling screening technique was utilized. In 2003, the investigation of the blood contribution for the West Nile virus resulted in the seizing of approximately 800 components of blood potentially containing West Nile virus [41]. In 2004, Macedo de Oliveira et al. said that NAT might not discern all virus-infected blood donors, permitting the transmission of the virus to continue at low levels [42]. They noted that assays of West Nile virus of NAT might vary in the sensibility, and combining samples improved the performance of the test [42]. The CDC noted six reported cases of transfusion-associated West Nile virus illness associated with blood component units with too small viral concentrations to be discerned by simple minipool NAT [41]. Macedo de Oliveira et al. said that discovery of the RNA of this virus by the contribution of individual NAT would be able to help show viremic blood that escaped minipool (MP)-NAT and maintain the transfusion-related transmission of West Nile virus [42]. In 2004, to improve the sensibility of the investigation of virus, blood collection agencies (BCAs) applied systems for switching the minipool NAT to individual NAT in areas with the epidemic spreading of West Nile virus [41, 43-44]. The CDC noted that clinicians should remain aware of the risk for transmission of the virus by transfusion of blood-products and official alerts to hospitalized patients with West Nile virus symptoms who have had a transfusion during the preceding 28 days [41].

In additional to blood donation, the organ donation is mentioned also as a new way of spreading the West Nile virus [45]. In 2002, Kusne and Smilack reported an identified infection of West Nile virus in the organ donor and in recipients of four organs [46]. In this report, the encephalitis developed in three of the organ recipients, and a feverish illness developed in one [46]. Three recipients came to be seropositive for the antibody of viral IgM; the fourth recipient had the weaving of brain that was positive for the West Nile virus by the isolation and nucleic acid test and the assays of antigen [46]. Kusne and Smilack proposed that organ recipients who receive immunosuppressants might be at high risk for severe illness after West Nile virus and transfusion of blood was identified as the probable source of the viremia of West Nile virus in an organ donor [46].

Genetic and Molecular Biology of West Nile Virus Infection

Genetics is an important factor affecting the ability of vectors to transmit West Nile virus. It is mentioned that variations in vector competence were controlled by one or more genes and expressed in variable proportions within a mosquito population [47]. Besides, the genetic basic parameters affect also the virulence of the viral pathogen. Beasley et al. suggested that glycosylation of the protein was a greater determinant of the phenotype of neuroinvasion of the mouse [48]. Brault et al. studied potential differences in the virulence of the raven with different types of West Nile virus [49]. In this study, American ravens were infected with old world types of virus of Kenya and Australia (Kunjin) and an American one (NY99) and it was shown that infection of ravens with genotype NY99 had a higher level of viremia in serum and death rate [49]. Brault et al. suggested that the genetic modifications in NY99 West Nile virus was responsible for the phenotype of virulence and that increased replication of this effort in ravens would facilitate the spread o fWest Nile virus in North America [49]. Genetic changeability and sensitivity of West Nile virus are also noted [50]. The gene of Flv showed resistance to the flavivirus-induced illness in mice for various different mosquito-borne flaviviruses, including West Nile virus [50-51]. Mashimo et al. recently reported the locality of resistance/sensitivity within an interval of 0.4 cM in the chromosome 5 that the authors appointed West Nile virus [52] and that corresponds to the region where Flv had previously designed itself [51].

The West Nile virus has a positive genome of RNA of a thread of about of 11 kb that codifies a single polyprotein [53]. Shi and Kramer said that the discovery of the RNA can be a new direction for the genetic diagnosis of West Nile virus [54]. Finally, Shi noted that inverse genetic systems of West Nile virus were very useful instruments to study many aspects of the virus, including viral replica, the pathogenesis, antiviral drug development and the vaccine development [55].

Pathophysiology and Clinical Manifestation

A. Pathophysiology of West Nile Virus Infection

The pathophysiology of West Nile virus infection in humans is largely unknown. After infection, West Nile virus replicates in the cytoplasm of infected cells [50]. Concerning the pathophysiology of West Nile virus infection, the virulence factor of the agent, West Nile virus infection, is an important factor. There are some studies on the virulence factors of West Nile virus infection. At the cellular level, Shirato et al. found that mice infected with viruses that carried the glycosylated protein developed lethal infection, whereas mice infected with viruses that carried the non-glycosylated protein showed low mortality [56]. In contrast, intracerebral infection of mice with viruses carrying either the glycosylated or non-glycosylated forms resulted in lethal infection [56]. Shirato et al. suggested that protein glycosylation is an important molecular determinant of neuroinvasiveness in the NY strains of West Nile virus [56]. Chu and Ng recently said that infectious entrance of West Nile virus occurred through the clathrin-mediated endocytic pathway [57]. In their work, double-labeling immunofluorescence assays and immunoelectron microscopy performed with anti-viral envelope or capsid proteins and cellular markers (EEA1 and LAMP1) showed the communicating pathway of internalized virus particles from early endosomes to lysosomes and finally the uncoating of the virus particles [57]. Destruction of host cell cytoskeleton (actin filaments and microtubules) with cytochalasin D and nocodazole showed significant decreasing in virus infectivity [57]. Nevertheless, actin filaments are shown to be essential during the initial penetration of the virus across the plasma membrane, whereas microtubules are involved in the communicating of internalized virus from early endosomes to lysosomes for uncoating [57].

In additional to the agent factor, the host response is another important factor in pathogenesis of West Nile virus infection. Biochemical and microarray analyses demonstrated that West Nile virus induced the expression of beta interferon (IFN-BETA) and several IFN-stimulated genes betas in contagion of cultured human cells [58]. Fredericksen et al. noted that the beta expression of these antiviral genes was due to the delayed stimulation of the transcription factor IFN regulatory factor 3 (IRF-3) [58]. Although the stimulation of the IRF-3 pathway was not sufficient to trap virus replication, Fredericksen et al. suggested that IRF-3 target genes work to constrain viral infection and limit cell-to-cell virus transmission [58].

B. Clinical Manifestation of West Nile Virus Infection

In the past few years, several large epidemics of West Nile virus have occurred in other regions of the world where this illness was absent or rarely occurred [18]. The infection is an arthropod-borne illness that causes a great variety of clinical presentations. The infections in humans are generally asymptomatic [4]. The most serious demonstration of the infection is encephalitis in humans and horses, as well as mortality in birds. Recently, nevertheless, a growing number of cases that imply demonstrations of the central nervous system and death have been reported in people of advanced age [4]. Fever, generalized body pain, headache, nausea and vomiting were the main clinical characteristics in an estimated 90% of the hospitalized cases [7]. According to the study of Weinberger et al., the participation of the CNS occurred in 170 (73%) of 233 hospitalized patients [10]. In 1997, Ceausu et al. studied the clinical demonstrations of 251 patients with this viral infection in an outbreak in Romania [59]. Ceausu et al. found diagnoses of West Nile acute encephalitis (166 cases), acute meningitis (57 cases) and acute feverish illness (33 cases). In this series, the most frequent clinical symptoms were fever (95.7% of cases), cephalalgia (92.6%), inflexibility of the neck (89.1%), vomiting (62.5%), asthenia (46.5%), and muscle aches (28.9%) [59]. In 2001, Weiss et al. reported the clinical demonstrations of 19 patients hospitalized with West Nile infection in the United States [60]. In this series, 11 patients had encephalitis or meningoencephalitis, and eight had meningitis only [60]. Severe weakness of the muscle in the neurological exam was found in three patients [60]. Fever and gastrointestinal and neurological symptoms dominated [60]. Weiss et al. noted that clinical manifestations in the areas of endemic or epidemic should be cause for a high level of suspicion during the summer in evaluating older patients with feverish illnesses and neurological symptoms, especially if associated with gastrointestinal complaints or muscular fatigue [60]. Conclusively, the reports of extraordinary, urban, and Western epidemics of Nile virus encephalitis in New York and Romania have indicated the exit of the neurological infection due to West Nile virus as a novel sanitary threat [7]. To document the frequency of this encephalitis, many researchers carried out a metanalysis of summative data previously reported [59-62] and found that encephalitis can be seen in 61.4% (197/321) of the infected hospitalized patients (Table 1).

Table 1. Metanalysis study to document the prevalence of encephalitis in West Nile virus infection

Study	Setting	Number of cases with West Nile infection	Prevalence of encephalitis (%)
Ceausu et al. [59]	Romania	251	66.1
Weiss et al. [60]	USA	19	57.9
Klein et al. [61]	Israel	35	10.0
Sejvar et al. [62]	USA	16	50.0

Wiwaniktit V, 2005.

Diagnosis of West Nile Virus Infection

Spread mainly by the nocturnal biting of *Culex* mosquitoes, the virus results in an infection that is most often asymptomatic or a feverish illness with limited symptoms [63]. Since most cases of West Nile infection present to medical workers with symptoms and signs of temperature, misdiagnosis can be expected. With respect to severe case with encephalitis, careful diagnosis is required, since the signs and symptoms of viral encephalitis are generally similar and they do not imply a specific causal pathogen. The routine cerebrospinal liquid exam revealed a common portrait of the viral profile of the infection [64]. CSF showed general pleocytosis, high protein and normal levels of glucose [64].

Several immune investigations for the diagnosis of the infection, meanwhile, have introduced both blood and CSF as specimens for examination. Neutralizing antibodies predominantly to West Nile virus could be discerned in samples of CSF by the method of 50% of the inhibition of the cytopathic effect. Instruments for measuring specific anti-viral antibodies in CSF that utilizes an ELISA test are also available. For blood specimens, there are various serologic assay methods for diagnosis, including immunoglobulin (Ig) M antibody-captures, ELISA, immunoglobulin G ELISA, antibody tests, tests of the inhibition of hemagglutination, and indirect fluorescent plate reduction neutralization test [65-66]. Nevertheless, the immune tests do not only permit the differentiation of another flavivirus in the group of encephalitis, including West Nile virus, in Asia and St. Louis encephalitis in North America [4]. Confronting this problem, there are recently developed immunoassays that utilize purified recombinant and non-structural protein of West Nile virus antigens [65]. Shi and Wong proposed that the non-structural protein 5 protein-based assay could definitively distinguish between West Nile virus and fever or St. Louis virus, as well as between the natural viral infection and vaccination [65].

Presently, molecular biology techniques are required for positive identification of West Nile virus [4]. Various instruments have been developed for identifying the infection, meanwhile, in CSF as well as in specimens of blood. RT-PCR is utilized to discern the genome of the virus in CSF and specimens of brain tissue. Guthrie et al. evaluated the use of RT-PCR for the identification of West Nile virus infection of the CNS by and found that RT-PCR well revealed the genome of West Nile virus in CSF and in brain tissue specimens [16].

Pathology and Complications

A. Pathology

Several pathological conclusions in the West Nile virus infection are documented. In 2000, Senne et al. studied the pathogenicity of West Nile virus in the model of chicken [67]. In the study, the chickens derived from a freed specific pathogen multitude were infected subcutaneously with a contagious dose taken from a raven infected with West Nile virus to observe the clinical signs and to evaluate the phase of viremia, microscopical and anatomical changes, the spreading of the contact, and the immune response [67]. According to this study, there were no observable clinical signs in the chickens of the virus-infected group during the three-week period of the observation, nevertheless, exam of histopathologic findings revealed myocardial necrosis, nephritis, and pneumonitis at five and 10 days postinoculation (DPI); moderate to severe encephalitis of nonsuppurative type was also observed in the weaving of brain of one of four infected birds at 21 DPI [67].

In the human, the majority of the infections are mild, as previously described. Nevertheless, the main modification in severe West Nile infection is in the neurological system, as already mentioned [59-62]. In 2004, Bouffard et al. reported an interesting description the histopathology of the brain and the spinal cord in infected humans [68]. They reported that an examination of the parenchyma of brain showed scattered microglial lesions accompanied by perivascular chronic inflammation and lymphocytic focal infiltrated leptomeninges [68]. The exam of the spinal cord showed lymphocytic infiltrates in roots of nerve and inside the appropriate cord, with focal nodules of microglial and neuronophagia in the horn ventrales [68]. Moreover, the special spots were refusals for a demyelinating process [68]. Bouffard et al. suggested the viral infection that was directed at the spinal cord and the nerve was established as the mechanism of flabby paralysis often observed in patients infected with West Nile virus [68]. In 2004, Guaner et al. reported another study of clinicopathological findings in 23 cases of West Nile virus infection [69]. In this study, lymphocytic infiltrates of perivascular spaces, microglial nodules, and the loss of neurons were predominantly observed in the brainstem and posterior horns of the spinal cord [69]. They noted that viral antigens could find the interior neurons and the processes neuronales predominantly in the brainstem and posterior horns [69]. Guaner et al. concluded that West Nile virus caused an encephalomyelitis by affecting mainly the brainstem and spinal cord and differences in the quantity of viral antigen could be related to conditions and fundamental medical length of survival [69].

In additional to the participation of the CNS, the West Nile virus infection is also mentioned for its participation in the eye. Khairallah et al. said that participation of the chorioretinal organ, frequently asymptomatic and limited, was common in patients with acute West Nile virus infection [70]. They noted that the extraordinary guideline of multifocal chorioretinitis in patients with systemic symptoms of West Nile virus could help establish the diagnosis, while a serological test was an alert; therefore, a systematic ocular evaluation, including a dilating exam of the fundus and angiography using fluorescein in chosen cases was recommended in patients clinically suspected of having this infection [70].

With regard to the abnormality in the profile of CSF, similar conclusions to other viral encephalitis disorders are noted [64]. The identification of West Nile virus Ig M in CSF is the recommended test to document the infection of the central nervous system, but this test cannot be positive in the complete spinal liquid less than eight days after the beginning of symptoms [71]. A series of CSF samples can be required to identify the antibodies [71]. Nevertheless, the persistence of antibodies of West Nile Virus IgM in specimens of CSF beyond 47 days was recently noted [72]. The researchers proposed that the presence of viral IgM might not always reflect acute infection with this virus [72]. With respect to the cell component in the CSF, Wamsley et al. studied 30 samples of CSF from horses with the infection [73]. They suggested that in horses with the beginning of acute neurological signs caused by encephalomyelitis, the findings in the CSF would probably be abnormal, mononuclear pleocytosis with a predominance of lymphocytes could be the majority of the commonly observed findings, and CSF of the lumbosacral region could be abnormal more often than CSF of the atlanto-occipital region [73]. Carson et al. recently proposed that a significant number of plasma cells in human CSF might serve as a useful early diagnostic indication for this encephalitis [74].

B. Complications

Generally, the West Nile virus infection causes a mild illness, called the West Nile fever, without serious complications [75]. The disturbances of the CNS are the serious demonstration of the infection. These neurological demonstrations can be encephalitis (very common), meningoencephalitis or meningitis [76]. Many complications due to the participation of the CNS in the West Nile virus infection are documented in medicine. Similar to other viral infections of the CNS, many sequelae in the neurological system due to West Nile virus infection have been reported. Ceausu et al. noted that altered mental status (89.2% of cases), trembling of extremities (40.4%), ataxia (44%) and paralysis (15.1%) could be seen as the sequelae in the West Nile virus-infected patient with encephalitis [59]. Acute anterior myelitis is also mentioned [77] and is believed to be the factor contributing to the additional flabby paralysis [78], a rare complication, such as stiff-person syndrome [79].

Hassin-Baer et al. noted that cross-reactivity among antibodies directed against West Nile virus and decarboxylase glutamic acid could have contributed to stiff-person syndrome development in the patient after the infection of virus [79]. Ceausu et al. noted that the mortality rate in West Nile infected cases was 15.1% in acute encephalitis, 1.8% in acute meningitis and 0% in acute feverish illness [59]. Klee et al. followed up on patients with West Nile infection after 12 months and found that the frequency of cognitive, functional, and physical symptoms was significantly greater at that time than in long-term findings, and included muscle weakness, the loss of concentration and confusion [80]. They noted that only 37% achieved a full recovery after one year and the youngest age at the time of infection was the single most significant prognosis predictor of the recovery [80]. Klee et al. said that efforts aimed at preventing the infection focus on populations of advanced age that are at increased risk for more probable and neurological demonstrations and more likely to experience long-term sequelae [80]. Similarly, Pile noted that older people were prone to develop the neurological manifestations, including potentially fatal encephalitis [63].

Treatment

The treatment of West Nile virus infection should be based on the severity of the infection. Similar to a general viral infection, the specific methods are not available for the treatment of West Nile virus infection [5]. Since most cases of West Nile virus infection are mild, no intensive treatment is needed in those non-severe cases. Nevertheless, supporting therapy is recommended for patients with encephalitis [5]. There are some recent reports on possible antiviral drugs for the infection. Morrey et al. recently carried out a study in cell culture and in rodent animal models to determine the efficacy of interferon alpha (IFN-alpha), interferon (IFN) inducers and ribavirin, alone or in combination with IFN, to treat West Nile virus [81]. According to this study, injection of intraperitoneal of IFN-alpha (qd for seven days), polyI-polyC(12)U (Ampligen every other day for seven days) and imiquimod topically applied (qd for seven days), administered one day before the viral challenge, were effective in protecting, respectively, 100%, 100% and 70% of mice from induced mortality by subcutaneous injection of the virus [81]. They also found that reduced mortality had a correlation with reduced plasma viraemia [81]. They noted that IFN alone or in combination with ribavirin in the virus-infected animal models might provide useful information for the subsequent treatment of human patients [81]. Jordan et al. reported another interesting finding—that ribavirin can be a cytopathic agent for West Nile virus replication and actually inhibited replication in neural cells [82]. They noted that a high dose of ribavirin was found to inhibit virus replication and cytopathogenicity in human neural cells in vitro [82]. At present, ribavirin is recommended as an antiviral therapy for patients with West Nile virus infection [83]. Additional clinical trials in humans are required for the development of antiviral therapy for West Nile virus infection. Although antiviral drugs are available for West Nile virus infection, the effective supporting administration can improve the result. In severe infection, treatment similar to that of other CNS viral infections should continue. Recently, Pyrgos and Younus reported successful high-dose steroid use in the treatment of acute flabby paralysis from West Nile virus infection [84]. Nevertheless, close control of the physiological disturbance during hospitalization and sequelae after discharge is necessary.

Prevention

A. Vector Control

The prevention of West Nile virus infection is the optimal method for controlling this viral illness. Since this illness is vector-borne, the control of the vector is important in primary prevention. Caution concerning mosquito vectors is important. Monitoring of the adult mosquito has provided information to local departments of health, i.e., the density, seasonal fluctuations, viral infection, minimum infection rate (MIR) and indirect data in the efficacy of the control of the larval mosquito after interventions or adult control [85]. For the effective control of *Culex* mosquitoes, integrated strategies vector control are recommended [5].

B. Vaccination

Similar to the infection of dengue fever, an effective vaccine against West Nile virus is not available. Although a few vaccines candidates are undergoing laboratory trials, no vaccine has been available commercially for the control of the infection in humans and animals [5]. Monath et al. noted that contagious technology of a clone is utilized to replace the genes that codify the pre-membrane (prM) and the envelope protein of yellow fever vaccine with the corresponding genes of the virus of the objective, West Nile. The resulting chimerical virus contains the responsible antigens for protection against West Nile but retains the efficiency of replication of the yellow fever 17D. Principally, the chimerical virus replicates in the host as the yellow fever 17D but immunizes specifically against West Nile virus [87]. Monath et al. noted that the technology of ChimeriVax led to rapid development of a West Nile vaccine, and the clinical trials could begin as early as mid-2002 [86-87]. In the horse, Ng et al. recently proposed for a Western vaccine, killed and new vaccine of virus of West Nile [88]. They noted that the vaccine was sure and efficient with 94% of avoidable fraction [88].

C. Rehabilitation

Rehabilitation is an important tertiary prevention for cases of West Nile virus infection. The main aim of rehabilitation is to limit the disability as the sequelae of West Nile virus infection virus.

Kunjin Virus Infection

Kunjin virus infection is a variant of the West Nile virus infection [32]. This viral infection was described as a variant of the Australian strain [32]. In 2001, Scherret et al. found that the virus of Kunjin isolates of Australia were antigenically homologous and different from the West Nile virus isolates of Malayasia [89]. Kunjin and West Nile virus are understood as a group of viruses narrowly related that can be differentiated into subgroups by genetic and antigenic analysis [89]. Similar results were reported in another study of phylogenetics by Correct et al. [90]. In the study, Kunjin viral illness was found to be endemic in the tropical parts of the Northern Territory and Western Australia, but has been absent in Central Australia since 1974 [91]. In 2000, the sudden occurrence of cases took place during exceptionally high rain in a succession of months, and the previous evidence of the activity of flavivirus in the endemic areas in the region of Kimberley of Western Australia was reported [91]. Gild et al. indicated the reintroduction of the virus to Australia and the establishment of local cycles of the infection with a progressive risk to the local population [91]. With regard to the clinical importance of Kunjin virus infection, this virus has been shown to be a causative agent of Australian encephalitis [92]. Since Kunjin virus is accepted as a variant of West Nile virus, the clinical administration recommended for infected cases with Kunjin virus is similar to that of West Nile virus infection.

References

[1] Guharoy R, Gilroy SA, Noviasky JA, Ference J. West Nile virus infection. *Am. J. Health. Syst. Pharm.* 61, 1235-41 (2004)

[2] Pauli G. West Nile virus. Prevalence and significance as a zoonotic pathogen. *Bundesgesundheitsblatt. Gesundheitsforschung. Gesundheitsschutz.* 47, 653-60 (2004)

[3] King NJ, Shrestha B, Kesson AM. Immune modulation by flaviviruses. *Adv. Virus. Res.* 60,121-55 (2003)

[4] Zeller HG. West Nile virus infection: a migrating arbovirus of current interest. *Med. Trop. (Mars).* 59(4 Pt 2), 490-4 (1999)

[5] Paramasivan R, Mishra AC, Mourya DT. West Nile virus: the Indian scenario. *Indian. J. Med. Res.* 118,101-8 (2003)

[6] Jamgaonkar AV, Yergolkar PN, Geevarghese G, Joshi GD, Joshi MV, Mishra AC. Serological evidence for Japanese encephalitis virus and West Nile virus infections in water frequenting and terrestrial wild birds in Kolar District, Karnataka State, India. A retrospective study. *Acta. Virol.* 47, 185-8 (2003)

[7] Thakare JP, Rao TL, Padbidri VS. Prevalence of West Nile virus infection in India. *Southeast. Asian. J. Trop. Med. Public. Health.* 33, 801-5 (2002)

[8] Malkinson M, Banet C, Weisman Y, Pokamunski S, King R, Drouet MT, Deubel V. Introduction of West Nile virus in the Middle East by migrating white storks. *Emerg. Infect. Dis.* 8, 392-7 (2002)

[9] Bin H, Grossman Z, Pokamunski S, Malkinson M, Weiss L, Duvdevani P, Banet C, Weisman Y, Annis E, Gandaku D, Yahalom V, Hindyieh M, Shulman L, Mendelson E. West Nile fever in Israel 1999-2000: from geese to humans. *Ann. N. Y. Acad. Sci.* 951,127-42 (2001)

[10] Weinberger M, Pitlik SD, Gandacu D, Lang R, Nassar F, Ben David D, Rubinstein E, Izthaki A, Mishal J, Kitzes R, Siegman-Igra Y, Giladi M, Pick N, Mendelson E, Bin H, Shohat T. West Nile fever outbreak, Israel, 2000: epidemiologic aspects. *Emerg. Infect. Dis.* 7, 686-91 (2001)

[11] Meco O. West Nile arbovirus antibodics with hemagglutination inhibition (HI) in residents of Southeast Anatolia. *Mikrobiyol. Bul.* 11, 3-17 (1977)

[12] Malkinson M, Banet C. The role of birds in the ecology of West Nile virus in Europe and Africa. *Curr. Top. Microbiol. Immunol.* 267, 309-22 (2002)

[13] McLean RG, Ubico SR, Bourne D, Komar N. West Nile virus in livestock and wildlife. *Curr. Top. Microbiol. Immunol.* 267, 271-308 (2002)

[14] Depoortere E, Kavle J, Keus K, Zeller H, Murri S, Legros D. Outbreak of West Nile virus causing severe neurological involvement in children, Nuba Mountains, Sudan, 2002. *Trop. Med. Int. Health.* 9, 730-6 (2004)

[15] Feki I, Marrakchi C, Ben Hmida M, Belahsen F, Ben Jemaa M, Maaloul I, Kanoun F, Ben Hamed S, Mhiri C. Epidemic West Nile virus encephalitis in Tunisia. *Neuroepidemiology.* 2005;24(1-2):1-7 (2005)

[16] Guthrie AJ, Howell PG, Gardner IA, Swanepoel RE, Nurton JP, Harper CK, Pardini A, Groenewald D, Visage CW, Hedges JF, Balasuriya UB, Cornel AJ, MacLachlan NJ. West Nile virus infection of Thoroughbred horses in South Africa (2000-2001). *Equine. Vet. J.* 35, 601-5 (2003)

[17] Garmendia AE, Van Kruiningen HJ, French RA. The West Nile virus infection: its recent emergence in North America. *Microbes. Infect.* 3, 223-9. (2001)

[18] Marfin AA, Gubler DJ. West Nile encephalitis: an emerging disease in the United States. *Clin. Infect. Dis.* 33, 1713-9 (2001)

[19] Bledsoe GH. The West Nile virus: a lesson in emerging infections. *Wilderness. Environ. Med.* 15, 113-8 (2004)

[20] Gould LH, Fikrig E. West Nile virus: a growing concern? *J. Clin. Invest.* 113, 1102-7 (2004)

[21] Power C, van Marle G. The emergence of West Nile virus in Canada. *Can. J. Neurol. Sci.* 31, 135-7 (2004)

[22] Gancz AY, Barker IK, Lindsay R, Dibernardo A, McKeever K, Hunter B. West Nile virus outbreak in North American owls, Ontario, 2002. *Emerg. Infect. Dis.* 10, 2135-42 (2004)

[23] Condotta SA, Hunter FF, Bidochka MJ. West Nile virus infection rates in pooled and individual mosquito samples. *Vector. Borne. Zoonotic. Dis.* 4, 198-203 (2004)

[24] Sayao AL, Suchowersky O, Al-Khathaami A, Klassen B, Katz NR, Sevick R, Tilley P, Fox J, Patry D. Calgary experience with West Nile virus neurological syndrome during the late summer of 2003. *Can. J. Neurol. Sci.* 31, 194-203 (2004)

[25] Durand JP, Simon F, Tolou H. West Nile virus: in France again, in humans and horses. *Rev. Prat.* 54, 703-10 (2004)

[26] Hubalek Z, Halouzka J. West Nile fever--a reemerging mosquito-borne viral disease in Europe. *Emerg. Infect. Dis.* 5, 643-50 (1999)

[27] Zeller HG, Schuffenecker I. West Nile virus: an overview of its spread in Europe and the Mediterranean basin in contrast to its spread in the Americas. *Eur. J. Clin. Microbiol. Infect. Dis.* 23,147-56 (2004)

[28] Lvov DK, Butenko AM, Gromashevsky VL, Kovtunov AI, Prilipov AG, Kinney R, Aristova VA, Dzharkenov AF, Samokhvalov EI, Savage HM, Shchelkanov MY, Galkina IV, Deryabin PG, Gubler DJ, Kulikova LN, Alkhovsky SK, Moskvina TM, Zlobina LV, Sadykova GK, Shatalov AG, Lvov DN, Usachev VE, Voronina AG. West Nile virus and other zoonotic viruses in Russia: examples of emerging-reemerging situations. *Arch. Virol. Suppl.* (18), 85-96 (2004)

[29] Ternovoi VA, Shchelkanov MIu, Shestopalov AM, Aristova VA, Protopopova EV, Gromashevskii VL, Druziaka AV, Slavskii AA, Zolotykh SI, Loktev VB, L'vov DK. Detection of West Nile virus in birds in the territories of Baraba and Kulunda lowlands (West Siberian migration way) during summer-autumn of 2002. *Vopr. Virusol.* 49, 52-6 (2004)

[30] Studdert MJ. West Nile virus revisited and other mosquito borne viruses of horses in Australia. *Aust. Vet. J.* 81, 56-7 (2003)

[31] Hall RA. The emergence of West Nile virus: the Australian connection. *Viral. Immunol.* 13, 447-61 (2000)

[32] Hall RA, Scherret JH, Mackenzie JS. Kunjin virus: an Australian variant of West Nile? *Ann. N. Y. Acad. Sci.* 951,153 60 (2001)

[33] Peterson AT, Vieglais DA, Andreasen JK. Migratory birds modeled as critical transport agents for West Nile Virus in North America. *Vector. Borne. Zoonotic. Dis.* 3, 27-37 (2003)

[34] Brownstein JS, Rosen H, Purdy D, Miller JR, Merlino M, Mostashari F, Fish D. Spatial analysis of West Nile virus: rapid risk assessment of an introduced vector-borne zoonosis. *Vector. Borne. Zoonotic. Dis.* 2, 157-64 (2002)

[35] Banet-Noach C, Simanov L, Malkinson M. Direct (non-vector) transmission of West Nile virus in geese. *Avian. Pathol.* 32, 489-94 (2003)

[36] Intrauterine West Nile virus infection--New York, 2002. *MMWR. Morb. Mortal. Wkly. Rep.* 51, 1135-6 (2002)

[37] Alpert SG, Fergerson J, Noel LP. Intrauterine West Nile virus: ocular and systemic findings. *Am. J. Ophthalmol.* 136, 733-5 (2003)

[38] Center for Diseases Control and Prevention (CDC). Interim guidelines for the evaluation of infants born to mothers infected with West Nile virus during pregnancy. *MMWR. Morb. Mortal. Wkly. Rep.* 53 ,154-7 (2004)

[39] From the Centers for Disease Control and Prevention. Possible West Nile virus transmission to an infant through breast-feeding--Michigan, 2002. *JAMA.* 288, 1976-7 (2002)

[40] Possible West Nile virus transmission to an infant through breast-feeding--Michigan, 2002. *MMWR. Morb. Mortal. Wkly. Rep.* 51, 877-8 (2002)

[41] Center for Diseases Control and Prevention (CDC). Transfusion-associated transmission of West Nile virus--Arizona, 2004. *MMWR. Morb. Mortal. Wkly. Rep.* 53, 842-4 (2004)

[42] Macedo de Oliveira A, Beecham BD, Montgomery SP, Lanciotti RS, Linnen JM, Giachetti C, Pietrelli LA, Stramer SL, Safranek TJ. West Nile virus blood transfusion-related infection despite nucleic acid testing. *Transfusion.* 44,1695-9 (2004)

[43] Dodd RY. Current safety of the blood supply in the United States. *Int. J. Hematol.* 80, 301-5 (2004)

[44] Custer B, Tomasulo PA, Murphy EL, Caglioti S, Harpool D, McEvoy P, Busch MP. Triggers for switching from minipool testing by nucleic acid technology to individual-donation nucleic acid testing for West Nile virus: analysis of 2003 data to inform 2004 decision making. *Transfusion.* 44, 1547-54 (2004)

[45] Update: Investigations of West Nile virus infections in recipients of organ transplantation and blood transfusion--Michigan, 2002. *MMWR. Morb. Mortal. Wkly. Rep.* 51, 879 (2002)

[46] Kusne S, Smilack J. Transmission of West Nile virus by organ transplantation. *Liver. Transpl.* 11, 239-41 (2005)

[47] Failloux AB, Vazeille-Falcoz M, Mousson L, Rodhain F. Genetic control of vectorial competence in Aedes mosquitoes. *Bull Soc Pathol Exot.* 1999 Sep-Oct;92(4):266-73.(1999)

[48] Beasley DW, Davis CT, Whiteman M, Granwehr B, Kinney RM, Barrett AD. Molecular determinants of virulence of West Nile virus in North America. *Arch. Virol. Suppl.* (18), 35-41 (2004)

[49] Brault AC, Langevin SA, Bowen RA, Panella NA, Biggerstaff BJ, Miller BR, Nicholas K. Differential virulence of West Nile strains for American crows. *Emerg. Infect. Dis.* 2004 Dec;10(12):2161-8. (2004)

[50] Samuel CE. Host genetic variability and West Nile virus susceptibility. *Proc. Natl. Acad. Sci. USA.* 99, 11555-7 (2002)

[51] Shellam GR, Sangster MY, Urosevic N. *Rev. Sci. Tech. Off. Int. Epizoot.* 17, 231 - 248 (1998)

[52] Mashimo T, Lucas M, Simon-Chazottes D, Frenkiel MP, Montagutelli X, Ceccaldi PE, Deubel V, Guénet JL, Desprès P. *Proc. Natl. Acad. Sci. USA* 99, 11311 - 6 (2002)

[53] Brinton MA. The molecular biology of West Nile Virus: a new invader of the western hemisphere. *Annu. Rev. Microbiol.* 56, 371-402 (2002)

[54] Shi PY, Kramer LD. Molecular detection of West Nile virus RNA. *Expert. Rev. Mol. Diagn.* 3, 357-66 (2003)

[55] Shi PY. Genetic systems of West Nile virus and their potential applications. *Curr. Opin. Investig. Drugs.* 4, 959-65 (2003)

[56] Shirato K, Miyoshi H, Goto A, Ako Y, Ueki T, Kariwa H, Takashima I. Viral envelope protein glycosylation is a molecular determinant of the neuroinvasiveness of the New York strain of West Nile virus. *J. Gen. Virol.* 85(Pt 12), 3637-45 (2004)

[57] Chu JJ, Ng ML. Infectious entry of West Nile virus occurs through a clathrin-mediated endocytic pathway. *J. Virol.* 78, 10543-55 (2004)

[58] Fredericksen BL, Smith M, Katze MG, Shi PY, Gale M Jr. The host response to West Nile Virus infection limits viral spread through the activation of the interferon regulatory factor 3 pathway. *J. Virol.* 78, 7737-47 (2004)

[59] Ceausu E, Erscoiu S, Calistru P, Ispas D, Dorobat O, Homos M, Barbulescu C, Cojocaru I, Simion CV, Cristea C, Oprea C, Dumitrescu C, Duiculescu D, Marcu I, Mociornita C, Stoicev T, Zolotusca I, Calomfirescu C, Rusu R, Hodrea R, Geamai S, Paun L Clinical manifestations in the West Nile virus outbreak. *Rom. J. Virol.* 48, 3-11 (1997)

[60] Weiss D, Carr D, Kellachan J, Tan C, Phillips M, Bresnitz E, Layton M; West Nile Virus Outbreak Response Working Group. Clinical findings of West Nile virus infection in hospitalized patients, New York and New Jersey, 2000. *Emerg. Infect. Dis.* 7, 654-8 (2001)

[61] Klein C, Kimiagar I, Pollak L, Gandelman-Marton R, Itzhaki A, Milo R, Rabey JM. Neurological features of West Nile virus infection during the 2000 outbreak in a regional hospital in Israel. *J. Neurol. Sci.* 200, 63-6 (2002)

[62] Sejvar JJ, Haddad MB, Tierney BC, Campbell GL, Marfin AA, Van Gerpen JA, Fleischauer A, Leis AA, Stokic DS, Petersen LR. Neurologic manifestations and outcome of West Nile virus infection. *JAMA.* 290, 511-5 (2003)

[63] Pile J. West Nile fever: here to stay and spreading. *Cleve. Clin. J. Med.* 68, 553-60 (2001)

[64] Wiwanitkit V. Cerebrospinal fluid examination and interpretation. *Buddhachinaraj. Med. J.* 17, 42 – 52 (2000)

[65] Shi PY, Wong SJ. Serologic diagnosis of West Nile virus infection. *Expert Rev Mol. Diagn.* 2003 Nov;3(6):733-41. (2003)

[66] Hazell SL. Serological diagnosis of West Nile virus. *MLO. Med. Lab. Obs.* 36,10-2 (2004)

[67] Senne DA, Pedersen JC, Hutto DL, Taylor WD, Schmitt BJ, Panigrahy B. Pathogenicity of West Nile virus in chickens. *Avian. Dis.* 44, 642-9 (2000)

[68] Bouffard JP, Riudavets MA, Holman R, Rushing EJ. Neuropathology of the brain and spinal cord in human West Nile virus infection. *Clin. Neuropathol.* 23, 59-61 (2004)

[69] Guarner J, Shieh WJ, Hunter S, Paddock CD, Morken T, Campbell GL, Marfin AA, Zaki SR. Clinicopathologic study and laboratory diagnosis of 23 cases with West Nile virus encephalomyelitis. *Hum. Pathol.* 35, 983-90 (2004)

[70] Khairallah M, Ben Yahia S, Ladjimi A, Zeghidi H, Ben Romdhane F, Besbes L, Zaouali S, Messaoud R. Chorioretinal involvement in patients with West Nile virus infection. *Ophthalmology.* 111, 2065-70 (2004)

[71] Roos KL. West Nile encephalitis and myelitis. *Curr. Opin. Neurol.* 17, 343-6(2004)

[72] Kapoor H, Signs K, Somsel P, Downes FP, Clark PA, Massey JP. Persistence of West Nile Virus (WNV) IgM antibodies in cerebrospinal fluid from patients with CNS disease. *J. Clin. Virol.* 31, 289-91 (2004)

[73] Wamsley HL, Alleman AR, Porter MB, Long MT. Findings in cerebrospinal fluids of horses infected with West Nile virus: 30 cases (2001). *J. Am. Vet. Med. Assoc.* 221, 1303-5 (2002)

[74] Carson PJ, Steidler T, Patron R, Tate JM, Tight R, Smego RA Jr. Plasma cell pleocytosis in cerebrospinal fluid in patients with West Nile virus encephalitis. *Clin. Infect. Dis.* 37, e12-5 (2003)

[75] Watson JT, Pertel PE, Jones RC, Siston AM, Paul WS, Austin CC, Gerber SI. Clinical characteristics and functional outcomes of West Nile Fever. *Ann. Intern. Med.* 141, 360-5 (2004)

[76] Horga MA, Fine A. West Nile virus infection. *Pediatr. Infect. Dis. J.* 20, 801-2 (2001)

[77] Gadoth N, Weitzman S, Lehmann EE. Acute anterior myelitis complicating West Nile fever. *Arch. Neurol.* 36, 172-3 (1979)

[78] Leis AA, Van Gerpen JA, Sejvar JJ. The aetiology of flaccid paralysis in West Nile virus infection. *J. Neurol. Neurosurg. Psychiatry.* 75, 940 – 1 (2004)

[79] Hassin-Baer S, Kirson ED, Shulman L, Buchman AS, Bin H, Hindiyeh M, Markevich L, Mendelson E. Stiff-person syndrome following West Nile fever. *Arch. Neurol.* 61, 938-41 (2004)

[80] Klee AL, Maidin B, Edwin B, Poshni I, Mostashari F, Fine A, Layton M, Nash D. Long-term prognosis for clinical West Nile virus infection. *Emerg. Infect. Dis.* 10, 1405-11 (2004)

[81] Morrey JD, Day CW, Julander JG, Blatt LM, Smee DF, Sidwell RW. Effect of interferon-alpha and interferon-inducers on West Nile virus in mouse and hamster animal models. *Antivir. Chem. Chemother.* 15, 101-9 (2004)

[82] Jordan I, Briese T, Fischer N, Lau JY, Lipkin WI. Ribavirin inhibits West Nile virus replication and cytopathic effect in neural cells. *J. Infect. Dis.* 182, 1214-7 (2000)

[83] Jackson AC. Therapy of West Nile virus infection. *Can. J. Neurol. Sci.* 31, 131-4(2004)

[84] Pyrgos V, Younus F. High-dose steroids in the management of acute flaccid paralysis due to West Nile virus infection. *Scand. J. Infect. Dis.* 36, 509-12 (2004)

[85] White DJ. Vector surveillance for West Nile virus. *Ann. N. Y. Acad. Sci.* 951, 74-83 (2001)

[86] Monath TP, Arroyo J, Miller C, Guirakhoo F. West Nile virus vaccine. *Curr. Drug. Targets. Infect. Disord.* 1, 37-50 (2001)

[87] Monath TP. Prospects for development of a vaccine against the West Nile virus. *Ann. N. Y. Acad. Sci.* 951, 1-12 (2001)

[88] Ng T, Hathaway D, Jennings N, Champ D, Chiang YW, Chu HJ. Equine vaccine for West Nile virus. *Dev. Biol. (Basel).* 114, 221-7 (2003)

[89] Scherret JH, Poidinger M, Mackenzie JS, Broom AK, Deubel V, Lipkin WI, Briese T, Gould EA, Hall RA. The relationships between West Nile and Kunjin viruses. *Emerg. Infect. Dis.* 7, 697-705 (2001)

[90] Wright PJ, Warr HM, Westaway EG. Comparisons by peptide mapping of proteins specified by Kunjin, West Nile and Murray Valley encephalitis viruses. *Aust. J. Exp. Biol. Med. Sci.* 61 (Pt 6), 641-53 (1983)

[91] Brown A, Bolisetty S, Whelan P, Smith D, Wheaton G. Reappearance of human cases due to Murray Valley encephalitis virus and Kunjin virus in central Australia after an absence of 26 years. *Commun. Dis. Intell.* 26, 39-44 (2002)

[92] Mackenzie JS, Broom AK. Australian X disease, Murray Valley encephalitis and the French connection. *Vet. Microbiol.* 46, 79-90 (1995)

Chapter VII

Rift Valley Fever

Epidemiology

Rift Valley fever virusis an endemic arthropod-borne illness causing *Phlebovirus* in sub-Saharan Africa [1]. Large epizootics occur at irregular intervals in seasons of above- average rain with persistent flooding and the appearance of many aedine mosquitoes [1]. Pretorius et al. said that epizootics of Rift Valley fever are often associated with periods of heavy rain, which is favorable for mosquito vectors; nevertheless, in seasons with normal or low rain, the circulation of enzootics has occurred, suggesting the existence of a natural host that would be able to act as an enigmatic bearer during interepizootic periods [2]. Outbreaks have also occurred in Egypt, in Madagascar, and in the majority of the recent cases in the Arabian peninsula [1]. There are many interesting reports on the epidemiology of the Rift Valley fever. Zeller et al. undertook a longitudinal study of the conservation of enzootics of Rift Valley fever virus from 1991 to 1993 in two areas of Senegal where prior evidence of the Rift Valley fever virus circulation was discerned, Barkedji in the bioclimatic Sahelian zone, and Kedougou in the Sudano-Guinean zone [3]. In this study, audits of mosquitoes, sandflies, and domestic ungulates were controlled with inspections of serologic parameters, and it was found that the virus of the Rift Valley fever could be cut off from the *vexans* species of *Aedes* and mosquitoes of *ochraceus* species of *Aedes*, but sandflies were not implied in the cycle of the conservation [3]. Zeller et al. concluded that the vectors of interepizootic appeared to belong to subgenera of *Neomelaniconion* in eastern Africa, and subgenera *Aedimorphus* in western Africa [3]. They proposed also that epizootics in eastern Africa were associated with an increase in rain [3]. In Egypt, a recent epizootic of the Rift Valley fever was reported in Egypt in 1997 [4]. In this epizootic, the signs among infected cattle and sheep were high fever, icterus, bloody and spotty diarrhea and abortion [4]. Abd el-Rahim et al. said that importing of infected ruminants, especially camels from Sudan, was the main source of the infection in the most nearby Egyptian province of Sudan, and was the focus of the infection of the virus in Egypt [4]. They also noted that the epizootics have generally occurred during the summer in Egypt as a consequence of high populations of insects [4]. Abd el-Rahim et al. concluded that occasional reoccurrence of epizootics indicated the failure of the vaccination program against Rift Valley fever in Egypt [4].

The recent spread of African Rift Valley fever to nearby areas in Asia is noted. There are some reports on the epizootics of Rift Valley fever in the Middle East. According to the report in September 2000, the first human documented cases of Rift Valley fever occurring outside of Africa in the Kingdom of Saudi Arabia and Yemen were noted [5]. They reported that this appearance beyond the African continent might be related to the importing of infected animals from Africa [5]. Due to the present-day globalization, travelers to endemic areas can be at risk for acquiring the illness if exposed to animals or their body fluids directly or by mosquito bites [5]. Special education with regard to both means of transmission and the geographical distribution of illness should be given to travelers at risk [5].

Vector and Transmission

With respect to the vector of Rift Valley fever, the virus is transovarially transmitted and can remain inactive in eggs of mosquitoes during dry interepizootic periods [1]. The circulation of a low level of the virus occurs in the high-rain wooded areas, although the individual cases of the illness are rarely recognized [1]. In a recent study by Pretorius et al., naive *Aethomys namaquensis* (Namaqua rock rat) were infected with Rift Valley fever virus and developed a viremia, but no clinical symptoms, suggesting that they could act as temporary asymptomatic carriers of the virus [2]. Pretorius et al. suggested a role for the rat as an enigmatic carrier of the Rift Valley fever virus during interepizootic periods and proposed a role as amplifiers, during heavy rain, for the Rift Valley fever virus circulation [2]. Anyamba et al. noted that all outbreaks of Rift Valley fever in Kenya from 1950 to 1998 followed by the irregularly high rain and periods of above-normal rain in eastern Africa were associated with the tepid phase from the El Nino/Southern Oscillation (ENSO) phenomenon [6]. They noted that anomalous rain caused floods of mosquitoes called "dambos" that brought transovarially infected eggs of *Aedes* mosquitoes that could transmit Rift Valley fever virus to humans [6]. Moreover, they proposed that analysis of historic data on Rift Valley fever cases and indicators of ENSO indicated that more than three outbreaks had occurred during tepid periods of ENSO events [6]. Anyamba et al. finally concluded that there was a close association between the changeability of the interannual climate and outbreaks of Rift Valley fever in Kenya [6].

Clinical Manifestation, Diagnosis and Treatment

In animals, Rift Valley fever is characterized by abortion in pregnant animals and a high mortality in newborn lambs and in calves [1]. Sensitivity to the illness is related to age and rises with severe illness occurring in the young of exotic castes of sheep and cattle [1]. For the diagnosis of infection in animals, several laboratory investigations are available. In 1997, Abd el-Rahim et al. carried out a virological and serological examination study for the diagnosis of Rift Valley fever [4]. In this study, several investigations in the laboratory were used, including remote virus identification utilizing a rapid agar gel test, complement fixation test, neutralization serum tests and the indirect assay of immunofluorescence [4]. They found that the tests of serological method yielded a greater rate of discovery than viral identification by agar gel and the qualification of the samples of the serum indicated that neutralization was more sensitive than complement fixation [4].

The virus causes severe hepatitis, especially in aborted fetuses and lamb newborns [1]. The illness should be differentiated from other conditions that cause death from hepatitis and jaundice [1]. With regard to the human infection, the Rift Valley fever is a zoonos, and human beings experience an influenza-like illness and, more rarely, complications such as encephalitis or retinitis [1]. In the recent outbreak in the Arabian peninsula [5], the patients presented with a feverish syndrome of hemorrhagic episodes accompanied by liver and renal dysfunction. Clinically speaking, Rift Valley fever is a fever of hemorrhagic episodes with hepatitis, similar to other hemorrhagic fevers such as yellow fever [7]. In 1994, Wilson et al. undertook a study retrospectively on the people who live in the northcentral part of sub-Saharan Senegal to investigate Rift Valley fever virus transmission to humans, with an endemic focus [8]. They found that seropositivity was similar for males and females, increased notably with age for both sexes [8]. According to this study, the risk factors for transmission of Rift Valley fever virus infection included caring for sick animals, helping animals during abortions/births, and treating sick animals [8]. Wilson et al. indicated that the disease was endemic in this region, people were at considerable risk for contagion, and that an up-to-now unrecognized method for human infection in non-epizootic conditions might be through contact with animals or infected humans [8]. McIntosh et al. noted that the majority of patients with Rift Valley fever for the most part were farmers, agricultural laborers and veterinary surgeons who acquired the infection during handling dead animals that had died of Rift Valley fever [9]. They also noted that some patients did not report a history of contact with infected animals and it was presumed that these cases were infected by mosquitoes [9].

Regarding the clinical demonstrations in human Rift Valley fever, according to a case of hemorrhagic episode that occurred in southern Mauritania in 1987 [7], various pathogenic syndromes in human beings, including an acute feverish illness, hemorrhagic fever, hemorrhagic fever with hepatitis, nervous syndromes or ocular illness were documented. With respect to diagnosis, techniques of laboratory investigation similar to those of animals are available. Diagnosis is based on the demonstration of antigen or viral antibody or by histopathology [1]. According to the report of McIntosh et al., the finding of an antibody response in serological tests could identify the most infected cases for isolation of the virus [9].

The complications of Rift Valley fever were common [9]. McIntosh et al. said that retinitis clinically associated with impaired vision occurred in about of 20% of investigated patients [9]. Nevertheless, the most serious complication of Rift Valley fever is central nervous system (CNS) participation [10]. In 2003, Al-Hazmi et al. studied 165 patients with Rift Valley fever and found that the greater clinical complications of Rift Valley fever included a high frequency of the failure of hepatocellular function in 124 patient (75.2%), acute renal failure in 68 patients (41.2%), and the demonstrations of hemorrhagic episode in 32 patients (19.4%) [11]. In this series, 16 patients had retinitis and seven patients had meningoencephalitis as a late complication in the course of the illness, and a total of 56 patients (33.9%) died [11]. McIntosh et al. said that in infected patients with meningoencephalitis, the pathology of the brain showed perivascular cuffing and round-cell infiltration [9]. Similar to other viral encephalitis diseases, the profile of CSF shows lymphocytes predominant with normal glucose and normal protein levels [12]. According to the registration data of the outbreak in April 2001 from the Saudi Department of Health, a total of 882 cases were confirmed, with 124 deaths reported [5]. Balkhy and Memish noted that the severity of the illness and the relatively high mortality, 14 %, might be a consequence of underreporting of less severe illness [5]. McIntosh et al. noted that the rate of mortality was high for the hemorrhagic fever with the hepatitis, reaching 36% [9]. The failure of hepatorenal systems, shock and severe anemia were the factors strongly associated with the patients' death [11].

With respect to processing of Rift Valley fever, a protocol similar to that of dengue fever infection would applicable in cases with presentation of hemorrhagic episode [14]. For cases with the participation of CNS, protocols similar to those of viral infections of the CNS should be utilized [14].

Prevention

Similar to other mosquito-borne infectious diseases, vector control is a basic method for primary prevention of Rift Valley fever. However, in animals, both an inactivated and a live attenuated vaccine are available [1]. New-generation vaccines are presently being tested, because of the reports that the existing effort of mousebrain-reduced vaccine induces teratology or fetal abortion in a percentage of pregnant animals [1]. For humans, the cloning of virus surface proteins that cause Rift Valley fever is in progress for future vaccination production at present [15].

References

[1] Gerdes GH. Rift valley fever. *Vet. Clin. North. Am. Food. Anim. Pract.* 18, 549-55 (2002)

[2] Pretorius A, Oelofsen MJ, Smith MS, van der Ryst E. Rift Valley fever virus: a seroepidemiologic study of small terrestrial vertebrates in South Africa. *Am. J. Trop. Med. Hyg.* 57, 693-8 (1997)

[3] Zeller HG, Fontenille D, Traore-Lamizana M, Thiongane Y, Digoutte JP. Enzootic activity of Rift Valley fever virus in Senegal. *Am. J. Trop. Med. Hyg.* 56, 265-72 (1997)

[4] Abd el-Rahim IH, Abd el-Hakim U, Hussein M. An epizootic of Rift Valley fever in Egypt in 1997. *Rev. Sci. Tech.* 18, 741-8 (1999)

[5] Balkhy HH, Memish ZA. Rift Valley fever: an uninvited zoonosis in the Arabian peninsula. *Int. J. Antimicrob. Agents.* 21, 153-7 (2003)

[6] Anyamba A, Linthicum KJ, Tucker CJ. Climate-disease connections: Rift Valley Fever in Kenya. *Cad. Saude. Publica.* 17 Suppl,133-40 (2001)

[7] Digoutte JP. Present status of an arbovirus infection: yellow fever, its natural history of hemorrhagic fever, Rift Valley fever. *Bull. Soc. Pathol. Exot.* 92, 343-8 (1999)

[8] Wilson ML, Chapman LE, Hall DB, Dykstra EA, Ba K, Zeller HG, Traore-Lamizana M, Hervy JP, Linthicum KJ, Peters CJ. Rift Valley fever in rural northern Senegal: human risk factors and potential vectors. *Am. J. Trop. Med. Hyg.* 50, 663-75 (1994)

[9] McIntosh BM, Russell D, dos Santos I, Gear JH. Rift Valley fever in humans in South Africa. *S. Afr. Med. J.* 58, 803-6 (1980)

[10] Alrajhi AA, Al-Semari A, Al-Watban J. Rift Valley fever encephalitis. *Emerg. Infect. Dis.* 10, 554-5 (2004)

[11] Al-Hazmi M, Ayoola EA, Abdurahman M, Banzal S, Ashraf J, El-Bushra A, Hazmi A, Abdullah M, Abbo H, Elamin A, Al-Sammani el-T, Gadour M, Menon C, Hamza M, Rahim I, Hafez M, Jambavalikar M, Arishi H, Aqeel A. Epidemic Rift Valley fever in Saudi Arabia: a clinical study of severe illness in humans. *Clin. Infect. Dis.* 36, 245-52 (2003)

[12] Wiwanitkit V. Cerebrospinal fluid examination and interpretation. *Buddhachinaraj. Med. J.* 17, 42 – 52 (2000)

[13] Isaacson M. Viral hemorrhagic fever hazards for travelers in Africa. *Clin. Infect. Dis.* 33, 1707-12 (2001)

[14] Shawky S. Rift valley fever. *Saudi. Med. J.* 21, 1109-15 (2000)

[15] Bachrach HL. Recombinant DNA technology for the preparation of subunit vaccines. *J. Am. Vet. Med. Assoc.* 181, 992-9 (1982)

Chapter VIII

Colorado Tick Fever

Colorado Tick Fever

A. Epidemiology

Colorado tick fever is an arboviral infection. It is also known as mountain fever [1]. This tick-borne disease is common to the Rocky Mountain region of the United States and Canada [1]. In 1974, McLean performed ecologic studies of small mammals in Rocky Mountain National Park in order to identify the specific habitats within the Lower Montane Forest that support Colorado tick fever virus [2]. According to this study, open stands of ponderosa pine and shrubs on dry, rocky surfaces were found to be important for maintaining Colorado tick fever virus [2-3]. Bowen et al. detected that the prevalence of infection in rodents was constant from April to July and then declined to 1.7–2.5% in August and September, coincident with a decline in nymphal tick ectoparasitism [4]. The involvement of porcupines, *Erethizon dorsatum*, in the ecology of Colorado tick fever virus in Rocky Mountain National Park was investigated from 1975 to 1977 [5]. McLean et al. found that porcupines utilize the same habitats described for the Colorado tick ecosystem in Rocky Mountain National Park and appear to be an important host for adult *Dermacentor andersoni* [5]. Indeed, population dynamics and host utilization of immature stages of the Rocky Mountain wood tick, *Dermacentor Andersoni*, is widely mentioned [6-7]. In 1982, Lane et al. noted that a virus very similar or identical to Colorado tick fever virus was recovered from the blood clot of one of 104 black-tailed jack rabbits (*Lepus californicus*) examined during a survey of various zoonotic agents in mammals and ticks from California [8]. This is the first reported isolation of a Corolado tick fever-like virus from *L. californicus*, and only the second time such a virus has been found in northwestern California [8]. In humans, Colorado tick fever is presently one of the important North American tick-borne diseases [9].

B. Vector and Transmission

The Rocky Mountain wood tick, *Dermacentor andersoni*, is the primary vector [1]. There are many interesting studies on the Rocky Mountain wood tick and transmission of Colorado tick fever. Eisen studied seasonal pattern of host-seeking activity by the human-biting adult life stage of *Dermacentor andersoni* [10]. In this work, densities of tick adults exceeded 50% of the peak when daily maximum temperatures were in the 16–19°C range and daily minimum relative humidity was > 20% [10]. In addition, tick seasonality may be adapted to local climatic conditions; site-specific daily maximum temperatures at the time of peak tick host-seeking activity in late April were positively associated with site-specific mean daily maximum temperatures for April [10]. Eisen et al. also noted that abundance of tick adults peaked at a mean annual maximum temperature of approximately 10°C and a mean annual growing degree-day value of approximately 650 [11]. In addition, relationships between climate variables and abundance of tick adults were used to create geographic information system (GIS)-based models for predicted tick abundance and indicated a shift toward peak abundances of tick adults occurring in sheltered northern/eastern exposures, rather than in drier and hotter southern/western exposures, at elevations below 2,100 m [11].

Transmission of Colorado tick fever virus is a vector-borne type. Transmission by this method has been confirmed for half a century [12]. In addition, there are also other new reported modes. Transfusion-related transmission has been reported. Leiby and Gill reported that because interactions between humans and ticks are likely to increase in the future, vigilance is required as new and extant tick-borne agents pose potential threats to transfusion safety [13]. Congenital transmission of this disease is probable. Desmond et al. studied the congenital Colorado tick fever in mice models and found that antigen or virus was demonstrable in only a low proportion of embryos, ill newborns or stillborns examined, but a high proportion of mice examined at a time when maternal antibody would be lost (6 and 12 weeks) showed antibody, indicating a higher incidence of infection [14].

C. Clinical Manifestation, Diagnosis and Treatment

The triad of high fever, severe myalgia, and headache is typical, but not specific. Although it is a self-limited disease in most cases, severe complications may occur [1]. In 1978, Goodpasture et al. reported a series of 228 cases of Corolado tick fever. In this report, although 90% of the patients reported exposure to ticks before illness, only 52% were aware of an actual tick bite [15]. Typical symptoms of fever, myalgia, and headache were common, but gastrointestinal symptoms were also prominent in 20% of the patients [15]. Zaidi and Singer noted that physicians evaluating patients who live in or travel to areas where tickborne diseases are endemic and who present with an acute febrile illness and gastrointestinal manifestations should maintain a high index of suspicion for one of these disease entities, particularly if the patient has received a tick bite [16]. Indeed, neurological manifestations of Colorado tick fever have been well documented [17]. Encephalitis can be seen in severe cases [18]. Paralysis can also be seen [19]. Persistent viremia (greater than or equal to four weeks) was found in about half of the cases; this finding was not associated with the occurrence of prolonged symptoms (greater than or equal to three weeks), which were also reported in half of the cases [15].

Considering the laboratory change in Colorado tick fever, there have been many reports. Hematological change in this infection is well defined. Significant neutropenia, as well as thrombocytopenia and a mild anemia, occurs in patients infected with Colorado tick fever virus [20-21]. Anderson et al. demonstrated that in the patients with Colorado tick fever, the mononuclear cell production of colony-stimulating factor was decreased and that there was an increase in circulating inhibitory factors in the serum of such patients [20]. The depressed mononuclear cell colony-stimulating activity does not appear to be reversible by addition of either endotoxin or normal human serum [20]. Characterization of these serum inhibitory factors may facilitate understanding of leukopenia in human disease [20]. In a recent study by Philipp et al., human bone marrow CD34+ cells and KG-1a cells, a human hematopoietic progenitor cell line, were infected in vitro with Colorado tick fever virus [21]. The time course and morphological appearance of viral replication in human progenitor cells were similar to those seen in erythroblasts and in HEL cells and suggest one possible mechanism for the clinical hematologic findings [21].

For diagnosis of Colorado tick fever, serological and molecular diagnosis can be used. PCR techniques have been developed that allow the diagnosis to be established from the first day of symptoms [1]. Recently, Calisher et al. designed an immunoglobulin M (IgM) capture enzyme immunoassay technique for the detection of antibody to Colorado tick fever virus in sera from individuals for whom diagnosis had been confirmed by virus isolation or neutralization test [22]. According to this study, although the neutralization test may remain the serological test of choice, the enzyme immunoassay for IgM antibody offers a simple and more rapid method of serodiagnosis; the enzyme immunoassay is, however, less sensitive than the neutralization test [22]. For molecular diagnosis, at present the knowledge regarding the genome of this virus is well established. Basically, Colorado tick fever virus, family *Reoviridae*, genus *Orbivirus*, contains 12 genes distinguishable by polyacrylamide gel electrophoresis [23-24]. Johnson et al. noted that the reverse transcriptase PCR method was a promising tool for the early diagnosis of Colorado tick fever viral infection, or for ruling out Colorado tick fever virus as the etiologic agent, in order to facilitate appropriate medical support [25]. Recently, Lambert et al. proposed a new quantitative real-time RT-PCR assay for the detection of Colorado tick fever viral RNA in human clinical samples [26]. This new quantitative real-time RT-PCR assay is efficient, sensitive and specific, and as such is useful for the detection of CTF viral RNA in the diagnostic or research laboratory [26]. For treatment, ribavirin may merit consideration in the appropriate clinical setting [1].

D. Prevention

Similar to other vector-borne infectious diseases, vector control is a basic method for control of Colorado tick fever.

Eyach

In 1976, an agent pathogenic exclusively for suckling mice was isolated from *Ixodes ricinus* ticks collected in a tick-borne encephalitis focus in Baden-Württemberg [27]. This pathogen is resistant to ether and sodium deoxycholate, but not to chloroform [27]. In the complement fixation test it showed a close, and in the neutralisation test a more one-sided relationship to Colorado tick fever virus [27]. Eyach virus, the pathogen of Eyach fever, can be isolated from ticks in France and Germany and is incriminated in febrile illnesses and neurologic syndromes [28]. This coltivirus is of concern at present. It is classified in categories A–C of potential bioterrorism agents by the Centers for Disease Control and Prevention [29]. Its ability to cause severe disease in humans means that these viruses, as well as any clinical samples suspected of containing it, must be handled with specific and stringent precautions [29].

Rocky Mountain Spotted Fever

Rocky Mountain spotted fever is a serious, generalized infection that is spread to humans through the bite of infected ticks. It can be lethal, but it is curable [30]. The disease gets its name from the Rocky Mountain region where it was first identified in 1896 [30]. The fever is caused by the bacterium *Rickettsia rickettsii* and is maintained in nature in a complex life cycle involving ticks and mammals [30]. Although it is not an arboviral infection, it is closely related to Colorado tick fever. For clinical characteristics, patients usually have a history of contact with tick-infested dogs and have fever as well as petechial rash [31]. Laboratory findings include high levels of hepatic aminotransferase, hyponatremia and thrombocytopenia [31]. Therapy with chloramphenicol and doxycycline is recommended. The mortality rate is high [31].

References

[1] Klasco R. Colorado tick fever. *Med. Clin. North. Am.* 85, 435-40, ix (2002)

[2] McLean RG, Shriner RB, Pokorny KS, Bowen GS. The ecology of Colorado tick fever in Rocky Mountain National Park in 1974. III. Habitats supporting the virus. *Am. J. Trop. Med. Hyg.* 40, 86-93 (1989)

[3] McLean RG, Francy DB, Bowen GS, Bailey RE, Calisher CH, Barnes AM. The ecology of Colorado tick fever in Rocky Mountain National Park in 1974. I. Objectives, study design, and summary of principal findings. *Am. J. Trop. Med. Hyg.* 30, 483-9 (1981)

[4] Bowen GS, McLean RG, Shriner RB, Francy DB, Pokorny KS, Trimble JM, Bolin RA, Barnes AM, Calisher CH, Muth DJ. The ecology of Colorado tick fever in Rocky Mountain National Park in 1974. II. Infection in small mammals. *Am. J. Trop. Med. Hyg.* 30, 490-6 (1981)

[5] McLean RG, Carey AB, Kirk LJ, Francy DB. Ecology of porcupines (Erethizon dorsatum) and Colorado tick fever virus in Rocky Mountain National Park, 1975-1977. *J. Med. Entomol.* 30, 236-8 (1993)

[6] Sonenshine DE, Yunker CE, Clifford CM, Clark GM, Rudbach JA. Contributions to the ecology of Colorado tick fever virus. 2. Population dynamics and host utilization of immature stages of the Rocky Mountain wood tick, Dermacentor andersoni. *J. Med. Entomol.* 12, 651-6 (1976)

[7] Eads RB, Smith GC. Seasonal activity and Colorado tick fever virus infection rates in Rocky Mountain wood ticks, Dermacentor andersoni (acari: Ixodidae), in north-central Colorado, USA. *J. Med. Entomol.* 20, 49-55 (1983)

[8] Lane RS, Emmons RW, Devlin V, Dondero DV, Nelson BC. Survey for evidence of Colorado tick fever virus outside of the known endemic area in California. *Am. J. Trop. Med. Hyg.* 31, 837-43 (1982)

[9] Wright SW, Trott AT. North American tick-borne diseases. *Ann. Emerg. Med.* 17, 964-72 (1988)

[10] Eisen L. Seasonal pattern of host-seeking activity by the human-biting adult life stage of Dermacentor andersoni. *J. Med. Entomol.* 44, 359-66 (2007)

[11] Eisen L, Meyer AM, Eisen RJ. Climate-based model predicting acarological risk of encountering the human-biting adult life stage of Dermacentor andersoni (Acari: Ixodidae) in a key habitat type in Colorado. *J. Med. Entomol.* 44, 694-704 (2007)

[12] Florio L, Miller MS, Mugrage ER. Colorado tick fever; isolation of the virus from Dermacentar andersoni in Nature and a laboratory study of the transmission of the virus in the tick. *J. Immunol.* 64, 257-63 (1950)

[13] Leiby DA, Gill JE. Transfusion-transmitted tick-borne infections: a cornucopia of threats. *Transfus. Med. Rev.* 18, 293-306 (2004)

[14] Desmond EP, Schmidt NJ, Lennette EH. Immunoperoxidase staining for detection of Colorado tick fever virus, and a study of congenital infection in the mouse. *Am. J. Trop. Med. Hyg.* 28, 729-32 (1979)

[15] Goodpasture HC, Poland JD, Francy DB, Bowen GS, Horn KA. Colorado tick fever: clinical, epidemiologic, and laboratory aspects of 228 cases in Colorado in 1973-1974. *Ann. Intern. Med.* 88, 303-10 (1978)

[16] Zaidi SA, Singer C. Gastrointestinal and hepatic manifestations of tickborne diseases in the United States. *Clin. Infect. Dis.* 34, 1206-12 (2002)

[17] Bartosik-Psujek H, Belniak E, Mitosek-Szewczyk K, Stelmasiak Z. Neurologic problems in tick-borne diseases--clinical and diagnostic aspects. *Przegl. Epidemiol.* 56 Suppl 1, 30-7 (2002)

[18] Draughn DE, Sieber OF Jr, Umlauf JH Jr. Colorado tick fever encephalitis. *Clin. Pediatr. (Phila).* 4, 626-8 (1965)

[19] Andersen RD. Colorado tick fever and tick paralysis in a young child. *Pediatr. Infect. Dis.* 2, 43-4 (1983)

[20] Andersen RD, Entringer MA, Robinson WA. Virus-induced leukopenia: Colorado tick fever as a human model. *J. Infect. Dis.* 151, 449-53 (1985)

[21] Philipp CS, Callaway C, Chu MC, Huang GH, Monath TP, Trent D, Evatt BL. Replication of Colorado tick fever virus within human hematopoietic progenitor cells. *J. Virol.* 67, 2389-95 (1993)

[22] Calisher CH, Poland JD, Calisher SB, Warmoth LA. Diagnosis of Colorado tick fever virus infection by enzyme immunoassays for immunoglobulin M and G antibodies. *J Clin. Microbiol.* 22, 84-8 (1985)

[23] Brown SE, Miller BR, McLean RG, Knudson DL. Co-circulation of multiple Colorado tick fever virus genotypes. *Am. J. Trop. Med. Hyg.* 40, 94-101 (1989)

[24] Knudson DL. Genome of Colorado tick fever virus. *Virology.* 112, 361-4 (1981)

[25] Johnson AJ, Karabatsos N, Lanciotti RS. Detection of Colorado tick fever virus by using reverse transcriptase PCR and application of the technique in laboratory diagnosis. *J. Clin. Microbiol.* 35, 1203-8 (1997)

[26] Lambert AJ, Kosoy O, Velez JO, Russell BJ, Lanciotti RS. Detection of Colorado Tick Fever viral RNA in acute human serum samples by a quantitative real-time RT-PCR assay. *J. Virol. Methods.* 140, 43-8 (2007)

[27] Rehse-Kupper B, Casals J, Rehse E, Ackermann R. Eyach--an arthropod-borne virus related to Colorado tick fever virus in the Federal Republic of Germany. *Acta. Virol.* 20, 339-42 (1976)

[28] Attoui H, Mohd Jaafar F, de Micco P, de Lamballerie X. Coltiviruses and seadornaviruses in North America, Europe, and Asia. *Emerg. Infect. Dis.* 11, 1673-9 (2005)

[29] Charrel RN, Attoui H, Butenko AM, Clegg JC, Deubel V, Frolova TV, Gould EA, Gritsun TS, Heinz FX, Labuda M, Lashkevich VA, Loktev V, Lundkvist A, Lvov DV, Mandl CW, Niedrig M, Papa A, Petrov VS, Plyusnin A, Randolph S, Suss J, Zlobin VI, de Lamballerie X. Tick-borne virus diseases of human interest in Europe. *Clin. Microbiol. Infect.* 10, 1040-55 (2004)

[30] Rubel BS. A case of Rocky Mountain spotted fever. *Gen. Dent.* 55, 236-7 (2007)

[31] Martinez-Medina MA, Alvarez-Hernandez G, Padilla-Zamudioa JG, Rojas-Guerra MG. Rocky Mountain spotted fever in children: clinical and epidemiological features. *Gac. Med. Mex.* 143, 137-40 (2007)

Chapter IX

Japanese Encephalitis

Introduction to Japanese Encephalitis [1]

Japanese encephalitis is a mosquito-borne infection. It is an infectious and non-contagious disease caused by an arbovirus, Japanese encephalitis virus [2]. Globally, Japanese encephalitis virus is arising as a more important viral encephalitis; alpha interferon was not effective against Japanese encephalitis in a double-blinded placebo-controlled trial, but new chimerical vaccines are in development [3]. Solomon said that recent work on Japanese encephalitis virus suggested that the virus originated in the region of Indonesian-Malaya, and in the extension of it there [3]. For a few years, significant advances have been made in understanding the natural history and pathogenesis of this viral encephalitis [4]. Similar to other pathogens that belong to the group of the arbovirus, the present focus has been in prevention by control of the vector [4]. This encephalitis can also surely be prevented by vaccination [4]. Mackenzie et al. noted that mosquito-borne flaviviruses, including Japanese encephalitis virus, provided some of the most important examples of resurging global illnesses [5]. Gubler said that there had been a resurgence and dramatic increase of arboviral epidemics, including Japanese encephalitis, affecting both humans and pets in recent years [6]. Zeller reported that air transportation permitted rapid transfer of illness from place to place and the diffusion of potential vectors or contagious hosts [7].

Today this illness still affects many humans, especially in Asia, and places a significant danger to unvaccinated travelers to these areas [1]. This illness can be classified as classical viral encephalitis. The infection can be diagnosed by serology, by the isolation of the virus, and by molecular diagnosis [1]. The illness is associated with severe encephalitis, a high mortality and a high incidence of neurological sequelae in survivors [8]. Japanese encephalitis is a zoonosis and it cannot be eradicated, but is avoidable in humans utilizing the Japanese encephalitis vaccine [1]. The true mechanisms of the illness of Japanese encephalitis were poorly understood and had not been the subject of modern clinical investigation. King et al. noted that members of the neurotropic serocomplex of Japanese encephalitis cause the functional changes associated with the enhanced efficacy of the immune response, in contrast with the majority of viruses which subvert or avoid the immune systems of host [9]. Japanese encephalitis was one of the illnesses causing the greatest fear of mortality before the development of an effective vaccine. Similar to other viral encephalitis diseases, there was no specific treatment, and the treatment of patients with the illness was very problematic, with the emphasis on the preventive vaccination. Nevertheless, Leyssen et al. noted that progressive investigation was identifying the possible objectives for inhibition, including the binding of the virus to the cell, the reception of the virus in the cell, the internal entrance site of the ribosome of hepaciviruses and pestiviruses, the mechanism that covers flaviviruses, the viral proteases, the viral RNA-dependant polymerase of the RNA, and the viral helicase [10].

Although have there been many efforts for decades to be get eliminate this illness, the infection still occurs sporadically. As a zoonosis, Japanese encephalitis cannot be eradicated, but the reduction of the human load of the illness is feasible by routine childhood vaccination in endemic countries, with a low cost when the benefits are taken into consideration [1]. Owing to globalization, Japanese encephalitis has become a contagious problem not only for tropical but also for nontropical countries. Bucens and O'Connor reported that while natives of endemic areas could develop the immunity, Western travelers were at risk [8]. Vaccination for the traveler is proposed for Japanese encephalitis [7-8]. Knowledge of Japanese encephalitis is, therefore, an interesting theme for general physicians throughout the world.

Worldwide Epidemiology of Japanese Encephalitis [1]

Japanese encephalitis is a mosquito-borne illness by arbovirus that is endemic in an extensive zone of Asia and the southeastern region of U.S.S.R. [8]. This illness is the most important cause of world epidemic encephalitis, totalling 40,000–50,000 cases per year [11]. It is limited to Asia, but its geographical area has spread [11]. Similar to many tropical mosquito-borne illnesses, the recent increases in the density and the distribution of the mosquito vector, as well as the growth of airline travel, has increased the risk of introduction and extension of Japanese encephalitis to the Western hemisphere [1]. A summary of some recent reports on the epidemiology of Japanese encephalitis in several regions of the world is presented.

A. Asia

Asia is the well-known endemic area of Japanese encephalitis. Southern Asia has the highest rate of infection in the world. In India, Kabilan et al. noted that Japanese encephalitis epidemics had been reported in many parts of the country [12]. They noted that the incidence had been reported as high among pediatric group with a high mortality, and the peak incidence of Japanese encephalitis in recent times has shown a growing tendency [12]. Actually, there have been many reports on the epidemiology of Japanese encephalitis in India. Kabilan reported that Japanese encephalitis was extremely endemic in the district of Cuddalore, Tamil Nadu, southern India [13]. Between July 2002 and February 2003, a pilot study was undertaken to examine if Japanese encephalitis was a component of pediatric acute syndrome of encephalitis (AES) in patients admitted to two large hospitals from the adjacent ones in Cuddalore, and to examine the distribution of the cases of this encephalitis [13]. According to this study, infection was established in 17 (29%) of 58 cases of AES; half were cases of AES (31/58 cases, 53%) and 59% of (10/17) of the cases of the encephalitis were limited to the Japanese encephalitis-endemic areas in the district of Cuddalore [13]. Kabilan concluded that in the Japanese encephalitis-endemic areas, the true load of encephalitis could be estimated by the collection of reports of cases of Japanese encephalitis in the local hospitals and of the reference hospitals [13]. In 2004, Chatterjee et al. carried out a serosurveillance to evaluate the frequency of antibodies to the Japanese encephalitis in children in various districts of West Bengal, India [14]. According to this study, the children up to 10 years of age in the four districts of West Bengal were in the part that had no immunity to Japanese encephalitis virus [14]. Chatterjee et al. proposed that if an outbreak occurred, the majority of these populations might be affected [14]. Kaur et al. reported an investigation of the Japanese epidemic of encephalitis of 2000 in Upper Assam [15]. They said that the epidemic was limited to the months of the monsoon that peaked in July and August and the case mortality rate was 42.11% [15]. They noted that there was no differentiation in the event between children and adults [15]. In this report, the male to female proportion was 1:0.6 [15]. Sehgal and Dutta proposed that Japanese encephalitis virus had caused many epidemics in different parts of India in recent years and should be classified as an important health problem [16]. Conclusively, Kabilan et al. proposed that Japanese encephalitis might come to be one of the greater health problems in India, about the significance of the vulnerable pediatric population, the proportion of Japanese encephalitis infections among the children with encephalitic illness, and scattering far from Japanese encephalitis-prone areas [12]. They noted that the load of this encephalitis could be estimated satisfactorily to some extent by reinforcing the diagnostic facilities for confirmation of this encephalitis in hospitals and by the conservation of contact with the nearby reference hospitals to stay informed of the details in cases of Japanese encephalitis [12]. Finally, Kabilan et al. said that vaccination was the best method to protect individuals against this infection and that it was essential to immunize pigs, a host that amplifies [12].

With regard to Southeast Asia, this illness is endemic in some areas. In Malaya, Sinniah noted that there was no program centralized by the Department of Health especially for caution and control of this encephalitis, even though Japanese encephalitis was endemic and sporadically occurs throughout the country every year [17]. Sinniah proposed that the drop of the discovery rate of the infection in Malaya might owe to the fact that the laboratory-confirmed cases represented only a small proportion of the total of all hospitalized cases that actually occurred, and another additional reason might be that these cases could not be confirmed by simple laboratory tests due to either failure to obtain a second specimen of the serum in the proper time or the failure to carry out lumbar drilling because of patient refusal [17]. Sinniah said that attempts to improve the rate of the discovery of cases of Japanese encephalitis in Malaya should be implemented to increase the clinical index of suspicion, instituting better procedures of the collection of specimens and adopting rapid diagnostic tests [17]. A similar situation in Indonesia was also reported by Wuryadi and Suroso [18]. With regard to the Philippines, Barzaga reported that Japanese encephalitis could be detected [19]. Barzaga noted that Japanese encephalitis occurred in the Philippines, with most cases affecting the 1–10 year age group in the places where fields of rice abound and the rate of morbidity was 15–17%, with a rate of mortality of about of 7–30% [19]. With regard to the region of Indochina, Okuno noted that the high incidence (annual rate of morbidity: 8.67–22.04/100,000) of Japanese encephalitis continued, as reported in the northern part of Viet Nam between 1969 and 1974, and a high incidence (14.7/100,000) was documented in the Chiang Mai valley, Thailand, between 1969 and 1970 [20]. Okuno also noted that the epidemic extended to the Chiang Mai valley and neighboring Shan State of Myanmar in 1974 [20]. After that, Japanese encephalitis came be a public health concern for Indochina. In Thailand at present, a recommendation for the vaccination against this infection for children in some specific areas such as mountain range of Phetchabun has been made [21].

In the past, Japanese encephalitis was known as an endemic, mosquito-borne illness in eastern Asia [20]. Wu et al. recently reported the epidemiology of Japanese encephalitis in Taiwan from 1966 to 1997 [22]. They concluded that the method of spreading remained the same as it had been: the phase of the amplification of the virus in pigs was followed by a human epidemic each year and, nevertheless, the frequency of the incidence of JE had significantly fallen [22]. They noted that the confirmed cases sporadically occurred all over the island and the distribution of the age of confirmed cases had gradually changed from mainly children to adults [22]. Wu et al. concluded that the change in the epidemiology might owe to program of vaccination, and the efficacy of the vaccine for those who received more than two doses of the vaccine, which was estimated to be about 85% [22]. With regard to Japan, the origin for the name Japanese encephalitis, the illness is believed to be eradicated.

Nevertheless, in 2004, Ayukawa et al. reported six patients who unexpectedly presented with Japanese encephalitis in early August to the middle of September in 2002 in the district of Chugoku, Japan [23]. They proposed that Japanese encephalitis in Japan was still a threat to adults and the elderly with diminishing or absence of immunity to Japanese encephalitis virus [23].

B. Africa

Although Africa is the endemic area for many mosquito-borne illnesses, it is not an endemic area for Japanese encephalitis. Recently, Fontenille evaluated the risk of introduction and potential amplification of various arbovirus diseases including yellow fever, Japanese encephalitis, Sindbis and Chikungunya in Madagascar, and noted that the risk was intermediate for Japanese encephalitis [24]. Actually, infection due to viruses similar to the serocomplex Japanese of encephalitis has been noted in Africa [25].

C. America

North America is not considered an endemic area of Japanese encephalitis. Similarly, South America is also not an endemic area of Japanese encephalitis. However, there are many cases of infections caused by Japanese encephalitis serocomplex in America. Therefore, surveillance for the possibility of new emergence of this disease is recommended.

D. Europe

Similar to North America, Japanese encephalitis is not common in Europe. However, the possibility of new emergence due to globalization has been mentioned.

E. Australia

Owing to close geophical proximity, Japanese encephalitis can be expected to spread easily from the southernmost part of Asia to Australia. Daley and Dwyer noted that Japanese encephalitis was an emerging new viral infection with a predilection for children in Australia [26]. Also, Mackenzie et al. recently noted that the Japanese encephalitis is an emerging virus in Australasia [27]. In the middle of January 2000, the reappearance of the activity of this encephalitis in Australia was first shown by the isolation of virus from three pigs from the Badua community on Torres Strait Island [28]. The additional evidence of the activity of this virus was revealed by the isolation of Japanese encephalitis virus from *Culex gelidus* mosquitoes of the Badua Pauls Island and the discovery of a specific virus that neutralized antibodies in three pigs in the community of Saint Pauls [28]. After that, human Japanese encephalitis was first reported in Australia in 2001 [29]. In 2003, Ritchie et al. studied the mosquito vector for Japanese encephalitis in the north pole of Australia and found that Japanese encephalitis RNA virus was discerned in 11/12, 10/14, and 2/5 pools that contained 200, 1,000, and 5,000 mosquitoes, respectively, utilizing a real-time TaqMan reverse transcription PCR (RT-PCR) [30]. Ritchie and Rochester proposed that regression analysis by simulation indicated that mosquitoes could have traveled airborne from New Guinea to Australia, potentially introducing Japanese encephalitis virus [31]. They also said that large incursions of the virus in 1995 and 1998 were tied to systems of low pressure that maintained strong northern winds from New Guinea to the Peninsula of Cape York [31].

Vector and Transmission [1]

Japanese encephalitis is a viral, tropical and important illness. This infection is an illness of arbovirus [1]. It is transmitted by the *Culex* mosquito; this neurotropic virus predominantly affects the thalamus, the anterior horns of the spinal cord, the cerebral cortex, and the cerebellum [32]. Schwarz noted that migration of humans and animals had been the path for the spread of viral illnesses throughout history [33]. In the Western hemisphere, for years, Japanese encephalitis has been diagnosed in travelers who returned from recent endemic areas [33]. There are some recent interesting reports on the vector of Japanese encephalitis. In 2004, an exceptionally high occurrence of *Culex tritaeniorhynchus* Giles living inside during the day was observed in a Japanese encephalitis endemic area, in Bellary district, Karnataka, India by Kanojia and Geevarghese [34]. Kanojia and Geevarghese said that increased endophilic resting behavior indicated that interior residual insecticides could provide an effective method of control in this area [34]. Another study by entomology method was carried out in Kerala, southern India, to identify the mosquito vectors of Japanese encephalitis virus and for determining its abundance and seasonal infection [35]. According to this study, Arunachalam et al. said that based on the high abundance and frequency of the Japanese encephalitis virus infection, *Culex tritaeniorhynchus* seemed to be the most important vector, while *Mansonia indiana* was probably a secondary vector [35]. In 2003, Kanojia et al. reported the long-term study on the abundance of vectors and seasonal frequency in relation to the occurrence of Japanese encephalitis in the district of Gorakhpur, Uttar Pradesh, India [36]. They found that the general population of the mosquito showed a bimodal pattern with high and short peaks during March and September, respectively [36]. Based on the density and the high infection with Japanese encephalitis virus, *Culex tritaeniorhynchus* had been considered responsible for causing the epidemics in the area. *Culex pseudovishnui*, *Culex whitmorei*, *Culex gelidus*, *Culex epidesmus*, *Anopheles subpictus*, *Anopheles peditaeniatus* and *Mansonia uniformis* were suspected to have some role in the epidemiology of Japanese encephalitis in the region [36]. In addition, the cases of encephalitis were reported between August and November with a peak in October when the population of vectors, especially *Culex tritaeniorhynchus*, were diminishing [36]. Kanojia et al. indicated that the anti-larval measures before the institution of paddy irrigation might verify the increase of vectors of Japanese encephalitis in the paddy fields [36].

Apart from mosquito-borne illnesses, the amplifying host is mentioned for Japanese encephalitis. In Asia, the pig is mentioned as the most important host that amplifies Japanese encephalitis [12]. The natural cycle of Japanese encephalitis virus in Asia implies water birds and *Culex* mosquitoes, especially *Culex tritaeniorhynchus*, with pigs being implied also as a host that amplifies and provides a connection to humans by its proximity to housing [37]. In 2000, Mwandawiro et al. studied the preference of vectors of this encephalitis in Chiang Mai, northern Thailand [38]. In this study, when mosquitoes were given a choice of being freed in a network that contained both animals, they exhibited a tendency to feed off the host to which it had been originally attracted [38]. The initial tendency of the vectors to bite cows was found [38]. Mwandawiro et al. suggested that effective control of Japanese encephalitis might be managed by enlarging the availability of cows (the no-way-out host of Japanese encephalitis virus) to deviate the vectors of pigs (the host that amplifies) [38]. A similar study was carried out by Van Den Hurk et al. in Australia in 2003 [39]. According to their study, in spite of the abundance of wild pigs in northern Australia, it was found that marsupials deviated the preference of host-seeking *Culex* far from pigs [39]. Van Den Hurk et al. noted that as marsupials were poor hosts of this encephalitis virus, the frequency of marsupials might hinder the establishment of Japanese encephalitis virus in Australia [39].

In additin to the spreading by vector, other means of spreading Japanese encephalitis are also mentioned. Some pregnant women can be susceptible to Japanese encephalitis, and if they experience Japanese encephalitis, the vertical spread of the virus to their baby can be expected. Intrapartum Japanese encephalitis is an interesting tropical. There have been no reports on the effect of intrapartum infection of this encephalitis on pregnancy outcome in the human; nevertheless, there are some reports in animal models. In 1981, Mathur et al. first reported the effect of the viral infection of this encephalitis in different periods of gestation in mice [40]. In their study, the infection during the first week of gestation caused a significantly higher number of neonatal and fetal deaths and in the number of abortions and premature births, and neonatal deaths were higher in infected mothers than in controls [40].

In this study, no congenital abnormalities were found in any of the mouse newborns [40]. In 1982, Mathur et al. reported transplacental spreading of Japanese encephalitis virus in consecutive pregnancies of mice [41]. They noted that the intra-uterine infection occurred in spite of the presence of antibodies of HAI against Japanese encephalitis virus in pre-conception mice [41]. Finally, Mathur et al. reported that the congenitally infected mouse babies responded poorly in all assays for cell-mediated immunity [42].

Genetic and Molecular Biology of Japanese Encephalitis [1]

Genetics is an important factor affecting the capacity of vectors to transmit pathogenic agents [43]. Similar to other mosquito-borne infections, it is mentioned that the variations in vector competence were checked by one or more genes and were expressed in variable proportions in the mosquito population [43]. Since 1987, the nucleotide sequence of the virus genome of Japanese encephalitis has been cloned [44]. McAda et al. found an existing homology between Japanese encephalitis RNA and protein sequences and those of the other characterized flaviviruses: comparative nucleotide (the amino acid) and the homological values for the M-E-NS1-ns2 segment of Japanese encephalitis were approximately those of West Nile virus, 68% (76%), and yellow fever, 50% (45%) [44]. McAda et al. noted that these molecular relations were in accordance with the relations of established serology among Japanese encephalitis and West Nile virus and it was disputed that these flaviviruses could have been diverted from a common evolutionary ancestor [44]. In 2004, Nabeshima et al. retrieved an acid amino as an attributable replacement to the acetylcholinesterase insecticide-insensibility in a vector mosquito of Japanese encephalitis, *Culex tritaeniorhynchus* [45]. They noted that the F455W replacement in the Ace2 gene was uniquely responsible for the insecticide resistance in the insecticide-resistant strain, the TYM mosquitoes [45]. In addition, vector resistance to the insecticide also depends on the resistance of the host to the pathogenic viral agent. In 1990, Miura et al. examined the resistance inheritance to the Japanese encephalitis virus using innate strains of mice [46]. They concluded that resistance to the Japanese encephalitis virus in the mice was checked by an autosomal dominant gene that was not linked up to a non-agouti locus on the chromosome 2) [46]. Finally, in 2003, Yun et al. retrieved a development and a possible application of a system of inverse genetics for the Japanese encephalitis virus [47]. They said that the Japanese encephalitis virus was an appealing vector for the expression of heterologous genes in a wide variety of cell types [47]. They noted that a reverse genetics system for Japanese encephalitis virus greatly facilitated the research in the virus biology of Japanese encephalitis and would be useful as an expression vector of heterologous genes and would help the development of a vaccine against this encephalitis virus [47].

Pathophysiology and Clinical Manifestation [1]

A. Pathophysiology of Japanese Encephalitis

The pathophysiology of Japanese encephalitis in humans is not fully understood. With respect to the pathophysiology of Japanese encephalitis, virulence is an important factor. There have been some studies on Japanese encephalitis virulence factors. At the cellular level, Su et al. said that during the infection of virus, the lumen of the endoplasmic reticulum (ER) quickly accumulates substantial quantities of viral proteins for the production of progenies of the virus [48]. In 2002, Su et al. showed that the infection of this encephalitis caused the unfolded responses of the protein (UPR) in the fibroblast BHK-21 cells and in neuronales N18 and NT-2 cells, in which Japanese encephalitis virus caused, as a result, cell death or apoptotic change [48]. They noted that Japanese encephalitis infection also led to the activated expression of CHOP/GADD153, a distinctive factor of transcription often induced for the UPR, and they appeared to cause the activation of p38 kinase mitogen-activated protein, an activator of posttranslational of CHOP [48]. The ectopic application of CHOP expression was related to virus-induced apoptosis, whereas treatment of Japanese encephalitis virus with a p38-specific inhibitor, SB203580, partly blocked the virus-induced apopotosis [48]. Su et al. concluded that emphasis on virus-induced ER stress might participate, via p38-dependent and CHOP-mediated pathways, in the process of apoptotic change caused by this virus [48]. In 2004, Lin et al. reported that Interferon (IFN)-alpha had only some degree of antiviral activity against Japanese encephalitis virus, in contrast to another flavivirus, Dengue virus serogroup 2, which was extremely sensitive to IFN-alpha in the cultured cell system [49]. They noted that this encephalitis appeared to yield the resistant cells to IFN-alpha since the IFN-alpha-induced luciferase reporter activity driven by the IFN-stimulated response element (ISRE) was gradually reduced as the infection progressed [49]. They found that the IFN-alpha-stimulated tyrosine phosphorylation of Stat1, Stat2, and Stat3 was suppressed by Japanese encephalitis virus in a virus replication and de novo protein synthesis-dependent manner [49]. Moreover, the Japanese encephalitis blocked the phosphorylation of IFN receptor-associated Jak kinase, Tyk2, without affecting the expression of IFN-alpha/beta on the surface of the cell. Consequently, the expression of various IFN-stimulated genes in response to IFN-alpha stimulation was also reduced in the Japanese encephalitis virus-infected cells [49]. Conclusively, Lin et al. suggested that Japanese encephalitis virus counteracted the effect of IFN-alpha/beta by blocking the activation of Tyk2, having as a result the inhibition of the of Jak-Stat signaling pathway [49]. Chang et al. said that Japanese encephalitis virus might cause acute encephalitis in humans and induce the severe cytopathic effects in various types of cultured cells [50]. In 1999, Chang et al. investigated which parts of Japanese encephalitis virus NS1 to NS4 were able to modify membrane penetrability [50]. They found that overexpression of NS2B-NS3, the virus proteases of Japanese encephalitis, permeabilized the bacterial cells to the B hygromycin, while NS1 expression did not [50]. In their study, their examination of the effect of NS1 to NS4 expression on the bacteria showed that NS2B exposed the greatest inhibiting growth rate capacity, followed by a modest oppression of NS2A and NS4A, while NS1, NS3, and NS4B had only an insignificant influence in comparison with the vector control [50]. They suggested that in the Japanese encephalitis viruses, these small proteins of NS hydrophobes had various modification effects on the cytoplasmic membrane permeability of the host, contributing in this manner to the effects of cytopathic viruses in the infected cells [50]. Recently, the studies using cryoelectron microscopy had characterized the flavivirus envelope protein as a new class of viral fusion protein (class II), and examined its arrangement on the surface of the virion [11]. Salomon said that changes in the envelope protein hinge region, or its putative receptor-binding domain, were associated with the changes in neurovirulence in the animal models infected with Japanese encephalitis [11].

In additional to the agent factor, the response of the host is another important factor in the pathogenesis of encephalitis. The role played by the immunized response in determining the result of human infection with Japanese encephalitis virus is poorly understood, although, in the animal models of flavivirus encephalitis, the responses of nonregulated proinflammatory cytokine responses can be harmful [51]. In 2004, Winter et al. studied the innate, cellular, and humoral immune responses in 118 infected patients with the Japanese encephalitis virus, 13 (11%) of whom died [51]. According to this study, these levels of IFN-alpha, the proinflammatory cytokine interleukin (IL)-6, and the chemokine IL-8 were all higher in the cerebrospinal fluid (CSF) of the nonsurvivors than of the survivors, both the IL-6 to IL-4 ratio in CSF and the level of the chemokine RANTES (normally T cell expressed and secreted) [51]. They concluded that during the infection of this encephalitis, the high levels of proinflammatory cytokines and chemokines were associated with a poor outcome, but whether they are simply correlated with severe disease or contribute to pathogenesis remains to be determined [51]. In 2004, Chen et al. noted that the induction of RANTES expression by Japanese encephalitis virus infection in the glia cells required the coordinated activation of NF-kappaB and NF-IL-6 [52]. Enzymatic inhibitors showed a strong correlation between the ERK signaling and RANTES expression; nevertheless, the virus replication of Japanese encephalitis was not dependent on the activation of ERK, NF-kappaB and NF-IL-6 [52]. They concluded that the infection of glia cells by the Japanese encephalitis virus provided early ERK, NF-kappaB and NF-IL-6 -mediated signals that directly activated the RANTES expression, which could be implied in the initiation and the development of inflammatory responses in the nervous central system (CNS) [52]. Salomon and Winter noted that the clinical studies had shown that innate immunity, as shown by the levels of interferon-alpha, was important in the Japanese encephalitis virus [53]. Salomon and Winter also noted that a failure of the humoral response was associated with the death of the disease caused by the Japanese encephalitis virus and the cell immunity had been less well characterized, but CD8+ and CD4+ T cells were thought to be important [53]. Finally, Ravi et al. executed an interesting study to examine the role of tumor necrosis factor (TNF) as a predictor in the infection of Japanese encephalitis [54]. They noted the elevated levels of TNF in the serum and CSF of patients [54]. They reported that this increase in the levels of TNF did not show a correlation with the duration of the disease, and an increased mortality rate was correlated with an increase in concentrations of TNF in the serum and CSF [54]. They summarized a correlation of laboratory parameters to the final outcome wherein it was revealed that the serum concentrations of TNF above 50 pg/ml significantly corresponded with a fatal outcome, while higher levels of viral antibodies (> 500 unities) in the CSF corresponded to nonfatal outcome [54]. Ravi et al. concluded that TNF can be used as a possible predictortor of a fatal outcome in the infection of Japanese encephalitis virus [54].

B. Clinical Manifestation of Japanese Encephalitis

Japanese encephalitis is an arthropod-borne illness that causes a great variety of clinical presentations, including a polio-like flabby paralysis [11]. The occasional symptomatic child typically presents with a neurological syndrome characterized by altered sensorium, seizure, and characteristics of intracranial hypertension [32]. In 1986, Le studied the clinical aspects of 116 children suffering from Japanese encephalitis B in North Vietnam [55]. In this series, the illness often appeared in the summer and affected 2- to 7-year-old children [55]. In the acute phase, the clinical portrait included meningeal signs, motor disorders, consciousness dysfunction and neurovegetative disturbances, and 90.4% of cases presented abnormal characteristics in the CSF [55]. Neuropathological examination revealed typical lesions in 16 cases [55]. In 1994, Misra et al. reported six patients with Japanese encephalitis [56]. They reported that central motor conduction time in the upper extremities was prolonged in three patients (five sides) and in the lower extremities in one (both-sides) that was consistent with the participation of the cerebral cortex, thalamus, brainstem, and spinal cord [56]. Misra et al. proposed that the changes in MRI and EEG in the acute phase might provide early diagnostic indications in patients with Japanese encephalitis [56]. In 1998, Kalita and Misra reported that the EEG pattern did not have a correlation with the Glasgow coma scale (GCS) and patient outcome [57]. They noted that an EEG with a nonspecific delta in the acute phase and the "alpha pattern" might be more common than realized, and does not always predict a poor outcome [57].

In Japanese encephalitis, seizures and an increase in intracranial pressure are associated with a poor outcome, and they can be potentially treatable [11]. Misra and Kalita noted that Japanese encephalitis associated with attacks in 46% of the patients in the acute phase of encephalitis is easily controlled by monotherapy [58]. They noted that the patients with severe encephalitis were associated with the highest frequency of attacks [58]. Solomon et al. suggested that in Japanese encephalitis, the attacks and the increased intracranial pressure might be important causes of death [59]. They noted that outcome might be improved by measures aimed at control of these secondary complications [59]. Regarding polio-like flabby paralysis, Misra and Kalita first mentioned this demonstration in 1997 [60]. They said that varying the degree of the previous participation of the horn cell was common in Japanese encephalitis [60]. Conduction of nerve and electromyographic studies indicated previous damange to horn cells in those cases [60-61]. Solomon et al. said that Japanese encephalitis virus caused an acute flabby paralysis in children that had similar pathological and clinical characteristics to poliomyelitis [62]. They noted that children with acute flabby paralysis in endemic areas should be investigated for evidence of Japanese encephalitis [62].

With respect to a predictor for outcome of Japanese encephalitis patients, the combination of coma, multiple attacks, and signs of brainstem illness for seven or more days are good predictors of outcome [60]. Misra et al. said that the best assembly of predictors of outcome included age, Glasgow coma scale and changes in reflexes [63].

Diagnosis of Japanese Encephalitis [1]

Most Japanese encephalitis cases present with symptoms and signs of encephalitis, making it difficult to do a diagnosis for the causal pathogenic agent. The basic principles in medicine, good history taking and physical examination, are necessary. Examination of CSF shows a result similar to other viral encephalitis viruses, along with normal glucose and protein profile [64]. There have been many current advances in the diagnosis of Japanese encephalitis. Microbiologically, the antigen of these encephalitis viruses can be detected in the CSF of the patients. It has been noted that antigen detection in the CSF is an inappropriate tool in the diagnosis of viral infections of the nervous system, especially in the first phase of the disease [65]. In 1994, Desai et al. examined 115 patients with a clinical diagnosis of Japanese encephalitis [65]. In this study, a test of inverse passive haemagglutination for the detection of viral soluble antigen, an immunofluorescence assay for cell-associated antigen, and an IgM antibody test were evaluated [65]. According to this study, Desai et al. concluded that diagnosis by antigen detection could be done less frequently than by the detection of virus-specific IgM antibodies in the vertebral fluid; nevertheless, antigen detection proved useful during the first week of the disease, when the IgM antibodies were not detected in the CSF [65].

Even with better laboratory options, the Japanese encphalitis virus usually cannot be isolated from clinical specimens, probably because of the low viral numbers in circulation and the rapid development of neutralizing antibodies [66]. Quantitation of this encephalitis virus by viral culture to contain the samples using susceptible cells is not applicable. Therefore, several immunological investigations are proposed for Japanese encephalitis. For many years, the hemagglutination inhibition test was employed, but this has various limitations in practice [67]. Principally, it requires paired samples of serum and therefore cannot provide a first diagnosis [68]. In 1980, antibody capture radioimmunoassay was developed [69] and continually progressed [70]; this soon was replaced by ELISA assay [71]. At this moment, the IgM-antibody capture ELISA (MAC ELISA) for serum and CSF has become the accepted norm for the diagnosis of Japanese encephalitis [71]. This assay is sensitive and specific; it is often positive for specimens collected on admission and distinguishes between the Japanese encephalitis virus and the other flaviviruses, including dengue, that are serologically cross reactive [67]. A new IgM immunoassay enzyme was recently proposed and was accepted as an alternate useful tool [67].

With respect to molecular diagnosis of Japanese encephalitis, there have been several attempts to develope a new molecular-based test for this purpose. However, most of the molecular diagnostic instruments are considered costly and not appropriate for the endemic areas, which are generally poor and marginalized. In 2000, Sun et al. noted that the period of toxemia of Japanese encephalitis patients was very short, so documenting the time of blood specimen collection would affect the rate of the detection of the virus [72]. They valued the viability of the RT-PCR for the detection of Japanese encephalitis virus: the sensitivity was measured by plaque formation test, and specificity of primers was proved by detecting some other flaviviruses [72]. They reported that RT-PCR was valuable in the diagnosis [72]. Huang et al. studied a TaqMan RT-PCR assay developed for detection and rapid quantification of the viral RNA of various strains of Japanese encephalitis virus [73]. According to this study, they found that the TaqMan assay showed a higher sensitivity and specificity than traditional RT-PCR methods as they had been previously reported and the application of the assay had been shown as sensitive for the detection of the Japanese encephalitis virus of both pools of the mosquito and Japanese encephalitis virus-spiking human blood [73]. Huang et al. concluded that the assay should be useful in the diagnostic conduct of the laboratory and could be utilized to replace or to complement the time-consuming viral culture methods, thus achieving fast, sensitive and extremely specific identification of the Japanese encephalitis [73]. Also, Yang et al. proposed that real-time RT-PCR assay that utilizes the single tube method could be used as a sensitive diagnostic test, and supplied results in real time for the detection and quantification of Japanese encephalitis virus [74]. As previously mentioned, since the majority of the patients with Japanese encephalitis are treated in rural hospitals with limited facilities, there is a need for an accurate and simple diagnostic test that is appropriate for such settings [67].

Pathology and Complications [1]

A. Pathology

Several conclusive pathologies in the Japanese encephalitis have been reported. The principal change is in the neurological system as mentioned previously [75-76]. In the animal model, Yamada et al. reported that nonsuppurative encephalitis could be experimentally induced in 3-week-old piglets by intravenous inoculation of either of two strains (IB 2001 or AS-6) of Japanese encephalitis flavivirus drawn from field pigs [77]. According to their study of the lesions, which consisted of neuronal necrosis, neuronophagia, glial nodules, and perivascular cuffing, they were scattered in the brain, the midbrain, pons, spinal bulb, and cerebellum, particularly in the gray matter of the thalamus and of the frontal and temporal thalamus [77]. In addition, Yamada et al. found that the antigen of Japanese encephalitis virus was immunohistochemically detected in the cytoplasm of the nerve cells in the frontal and temporal lobe of the cerebrum and in the gray matter of the thalamus and midbrain [77].

In the human, Prakash et al. used diffusion-weighted imaging (DWI) in making the diagnosis of Japanese encephalitis and the characteristic engagement found bilaterally in the thalamus [78]. In 2000, Kalita and Misra studied the conclusions of MRI in the diagnosis of 31 cases of Japanese encephalitis [78]. According to this study, MRI revealed either mixed intensity or hypointense lesion on T (1) and hyperintense or mixed intensity lesion on T (2) in the thalamus in all but two patients [79]. Abnormal MRI was also noted in the basal ganglions in 11, the midbrain in 18, the pons in eight, the cerebellum and the cerebral cortex in each of six patients, and subcortical white matter in two patients [79]. In additional to the pathology of the thalamus, abnormalities in the other areas of the CNS in cases of Japanese encephalitis also are presented. Pradhan et al. said that some patients with Japanese encephalitis could have lesions predominantly in the substantia nigra [80]. They also reported that after recovery from encephalitic illness, these cases usually demonstrated typical clinical parkinsonian characteristics [80]. In additional to brain lesions, the involvement of anterior horn cells can be found, as previously mentioned [11, 60].

With regard to abmormalities in the CSF profile, similarities to viral encephalitis are noted [64]. Johnson et al. studied the CSF in 15 cases of Japanese encephalitis [81]. According to this study, they noted that in the CSF of patients with Japanese encephalitis, the T cells dominated with a proportion of 4.2:1 of helper/inducer T to the suppressor/cytotoxic T cells; the B cells and the macrophages were often present, but in small numbers compared to their presence in the blood [81]. They also noted that cell type distribution did not vary between the first and last day of hospitalization, was similar in fatal and nonfatal, and was not affected by the administration of steroids [81]. Sato et al. noted that among atypical lymphocytes (AL) morphologically and immunohistochemically examined in the CSF of adult patients with encephalitis, a CD4 + "type I" AL with a multilobulated nucleus that seemed similar to the abnormal cells in the adult leukemia T-cells, could distinguish a CD8 + "type II" AL, a large lymphocyte with basophilic cytoplasm and a nucleus that contained rough chromatin [82].

B. Complications

Many complications of Japanese encephalitis are reported in medicine. Similar to other encephalitis viruses, a large number of neurological sequelae from Japanese encephalitis have been reported. Changes in electroencephalograph (EEG) and seizures are common complications. Kalita and Misra said that the model of EEG did not correspond to the GCS and the outcome in patients with encephalitis and EEG revealed that a non-specific delta in the acute stage and "alpha pattern" coma could be a more common presentation than previously realized and did not always predict a poor outcome [57]. In 1993, Kumar et al. studied the sequelae of clinical Japanese encephalitis in children [83]. In this study, a high rate of major sequelae (45.5%) in the form of frank motor deficits (32.7%), mental retardation (21.8%) and convulsions (18.2%) was observed [83]. In addition 25.4% had minor deficits only in the form of a scholastic delay, behavioral problems and/or subtle neurological signs and only 29.2% patients were completely normal on follow up [83]. According to this study, Kumar et al. noted that the neurological deficits were various and improved even after two years of the disease, and complications of the disease were harsher if the initial disease was extended,or was associated with focal neurological deficits [83].

Regarding cases with substantia nigra lesions, Parkinsonism as an important complication should be noted [80, 84]. In the view of neuropsychiatry, behavioral changes following Japanese encephalitis should be a concern [85]. Monnet said this pyramid-shaped syndrome, Parkinsonism and amnesia were the most significant acute deficits [86]. Monnet reported that whereas these faded in great part during convalescence, emotional instability and associated behavior with emotional engagement, obsessive compulsive symptoms and the cognitive disturbances appeared [86]. Monnet also noted that a partial recovery was attained with neuroleptics, lithium and the electroshock therapy [86].

In additional to common neurological sequelae, some rare conditions also are mentioned. In 2004, Hamano et al. reported a case of severe motor impairment and intellectual disabilities from Japanese encephalitis sequelae [87]. In this report, a case of Japanese encephalitis showed repeated vocal cord abductor disturbance due to laryngeal dystonia, in addition to generalized dystonia, in whom MRI revealed basal ganglia lesions; tracheostomy was effective for this case [87].

Treatment [1]

The treatment of Japanese encephalitis should be based on the severity of the infection. Similar to general viral infection, the specific treatment plays a minor role in Japanese encephalitis. A specific antiviral drug is not available at this moment. There are some recent reports on possible antiviral drugs for Japanese encephalitis viral infection. In 2003, Salomon et al. evaluated the efficacy of interferon alpha-2a in Japanese encephalitis [88]. They did a randomized double-blind placebo-controlled trial of interferon alpha-2a (10 million units/m^2, daily for seven days) in 112 Vietnamese children with presumed Japanese encephalitis, 87 of whom had serologically confirmed infections, and the final primary outcomes were death in hospitals or harsh sequelae [88]. According to this study, outcome at discharge and three months later did not differ between the two treatment groups; 20 children in the interferon group had a poor outcome, compared with 18 in the placebo group; there was no secondary effect of long-term use of interferon [88]. Salomon et al. concluded that the doses of interferon alpha-2a given in this regimen did not improve the results of treatment in the patients with Japanese encephalitis [88]. In 2003, Saxena et al. studied the infection inhibition of Japanese encephalitis viruses by diethyldithiocarbamate, a low molecular weight dithiol [89]. In this work, they showed that the production of nitric oxide (NO) through the activity induction of iNOS was meditated while circulating macrophage-derived factor (MDF), which could be responsible for the delayed progression of the disease [89]. They noted that DDTC-mediated inhibition of Japanese encephalitis virus was believed to involve the augmentation of the protective role of MDF, as evidenced by the observation that this pretreatment with the anti-MDF antibody significantly diminished the AST of mice, together with the inhibition of ion activity [89]. Sabena et al. concluded that DDTC could have a possible therapeutic role during the infection of Japanese encephalitis [89]. Although no antiviral drug is available against Japanese encephalitis, effective therapy can improve the outcome [32]. The standard protocol for viral encephalitis care [90] should be followed. Careful monitoring of psychological disturbances during the hospitalization and sequelae after discharge is necessary.

Prevention [1]

A. Vector Control

The prevention of Japanese encephalitis is a good method for controlling this viral illness. Since this illness is spread by vector, control of the vector is important in primary prevention. The classical methods, such as insecticide and bed nets, are requested extensively in the endemic areas [32]. Nevertheless, the most effective method for the prevention of this encephalitis is vaccination.

B. Vaccination [91]

Similar to yellow fever, an effective vaccine for Japanese encephalitis was developed a long time ago. A safe, effective, formalin-inactivated vaccine against Japanese encephalitis has been available for many years. This vaccine has shown its effectiveness for the control of Japanese encephalitis. However, it is still an expensive vaccine. A less expensive, live and newer vaccine is therefore under development. A chimerical vaccine of which Japanese encephalitis structural proteins are inserted into the 17D yellow fever vaccine structure is one of several vaccines in the development [37].

Kabilan noted that since the control of Japanese encephalitis by means of vector control were limited to the sustainability and the cost efficiency of the programs, the viability of Japanese encephalitis vaccination in India had to be considered as a preventive measure, in which identification of risk areas, target populations to be immunized, and cost evaluation of immunization are emphasized [92]. Generally, Japanese encephalitis vaccine is a live attenuated vaccine of virus by-product of infected mouse brain with Thimerosal added as a preservative [93]. The studies show this vaccine to be 70%–97% effective in preventing the illness [93]. The dose recommended for people three years of age is three doses of 1.0 mL subcutaneously and the primary series recommended for the immunization is given in 0, 7, and 30 days [21, 93]. For children aged one to three years, a series of three doses of 0.5 mL should be given in 0, 7, 30 days [21, 93]. There is no information on the efficacy and the security of vaccine in children under one year of age and the pregnant women; vaccination should differ in these cases. Vaccination for individuals with the symptomatic infection of HIV is still controversial. More studies on this topic are recommended. The vaccination is recommended also before travelling to the endemic countries [7]. This vaccination remains important in travel medicine [7, 94]. The vaccine of Japanese encephalitis is recommended for people who plan to reside for a month or longer in areas where Japanese encephalitis virus is endemic or epidemic [93-94]. Depending on the circumstances of the epidemic, the vaccine should be considered for people who spend less than 30 days whose activities, such as extensive outdoor activities in rural areas, place them at especially high risk for the exposure [93]. Lo and Gluckman concluded that Japanese encephalitis vaccine should be offered to travelers who plan prolonged visits to rural areas in Southeast Asia or India during the spreading season [95]. A shortened vaccination schedule of 0, 7, and 14 days can be utilized when the longest schedule is impractical due to limitations of time, but the last dose should be given at least 10 days before beginning an international trip to ensure an immune response and adequate access to medical care in case of a delayed adverse reaction [93].

With regard to adverse events of Japanese encephalitis vaccination, allergy to the vaccine has been mentioned [96]. Plesner et al. found that about a third of the adverse reactions to the Japanese encephalitis vaccine could be attributed to an allergic predisposition to the vaccine [97]. They said that the main factors of risk were young age, female gender and prior skin reactions or allergy to pollen [97]. Plesner et al. concluded that information concerning any history of allergy in young adults should be given before vaccination, the vaccination should be carried out more than a week before leaving and treatment with antihistamines should be available if a reaction occurs [97]. Severe allergy or anaphylaxis is also documented [98]. Sakaguchi and Inouye noted that two patterns of systemic immediate-type reactions to

Japanese encephalitis vaccines can be found: one with presentation accompanied by respiratory and cutaneous symptoms and the other accompanied by cardiovascular symptoms without respiratory or cutaneous symptoms [99]. They found that the children in the previous group had anti-gelatin IgE in their sera, whereas those in the latter group did not [99]. In addition to allergy, there are other adverse effects, rarely reported. Meningoencephalitis [100] and syndrome of Gianotti-Crosti [101] are examples. Similar to yellow fever, although there are reports of adverse effects from the vaccinations, the risk to non-immunized individuals who to live in or travel to areas where there is known spread of Japanese encephalitis is far greater than the risk of having a vaccine-related adverse effect.

C. Rehabilitation

Rehabilitation is an important tertiary prevention for cases of Japanese encephalitis. The main aim of the rehabilitation is to limit the disabilities that result from the sequelae of Japanese encephalitis virus infection.

References

[1] Wiwanitkit V. Japanese encephalitis. *J. Ped. Infect. Dis.* 2, 183 – 92 (2007)

[2] Halstead SB, Jacobson J. Japanese encephalitis. *Adv. Virus. Res.* 61, 103-38 (2003)

[3] Solomon T. Exotic and emerging viral encephalitides. *Curr. Opin. Neurol.* 16, 411-8 (2003)

[4] Whitley RJ, Gnann JW. Viral encephalitis: familiar infections and emerging pathogens. *Lancet.* 359, 507-13 (2002)

[5] Mackenzie JS, Gubler DJ, Petersen LR. Emerging flaviviruses: the spread and resurgence of Japanese encephalitis, West Nile and dengue viruses. *Nat. Med.* 10(12 Suppl), S98-S109 (2004)

[6] Gubler DJ. The global emergence/resurgence of arboviral diseases as public health problems. *Arch. Med. Res.* 33, 330-42 (2002)

[7] Zeller HG. Dengue, arbovirus and migrations in the Indian Ocean. *Bull. Soc. Pathol. Exot.* 91, 56-60 (1998)

[8] Bucens M, O'Connor L. Japanese encephalitis and the traveller. *Aust. Fam. Physician.* 19, 163-5 (1990)

[9] King NJ, Shrestha B, Kesson AM. Immune modulation by flaviviruses. *Adv. Virus. Res.* 60, 121-55 (2003)

[10] Leyssen P, De Clercq E, Neyts J. Perspectives for the treatment of infections with Flaviviridae. *Clin. Microbiol. Rev.* 13, 67-82 (2000)

[11] Solomon T. Recent advances in Japanese encephalitis. *J. Neurovirol.* 9, 274-83 (2003)

[12] Kabilan L, Rajendran R, Arunachalam N, Ramesh S, Srinivasan S, Samuel PP, Dash AP. Japanese encephalitis in India: an overview. *Indian. J. Pediatr.* 71, 609-15 (2004)

[13] Kabilan L, Vrati S, Ramesh S, Srinivasan S, Appaiahgari MB, Arunachalam N, Thenmozhi V, Kumaravel SM, Samuel PP, Rajendran R. Japanese encephalitis virus

(JEV) is an important cause of encephalitis among children in Cuddalore district, Tamil Nadu, India. *J. Clin. Virol.* 31, 153-9 (2004)

[14] Chatterjee S, Chattopadhyay D, Bhattacharya MK, Mukherjee B. Serosurveillance for Japanese encephalitis in children in several districts of West Bengal, India. *Acta. Paediatr.* 93, 390-3 (2004)

[15] Kaur R, Agarwal CS, Das D. An investigation into the JE epidemic of 2000 in Upper Assam--a perspective study. *J. Commun. Dis.* 34,135-45 (2002)

[16] Sehgal A, Dutta AK. Changing perspectives in Japanese encephalitis in India. *Trop. Doct.* 33, 131-4 (2003)

[17] Sinniah M. A review of Japanese-B virus encephalitis in Malaysia. *Southeast. Asian. J. Trop. Med. Public. Health.* 20, 581-5 (1989)

[18] Wuryadi S, Suroso T. Japanese encephalitis in Indonesia. *Southeast. Asian. J. Trop. Med. Public. Health.* 20, 575-80 (1989)

[19] Barzaga NG. A review of Japanese encephalitis cases in the Philippines (1972-1985). *Southeast. Asian. J. Trop. Med. Public. Health.* 20, 587-92 (1989)

[20] Okuno T. An epidemiological review of Japanese encephalitis. *World. Health. Stat. Q.* 31, 120-33 (1978)

[21] Wiwanitkit V. Consideration in immunization in the present day. *Taksin. Med. J.* 22, 250 – 3 (2001)

[22] Wu YC, Huang YS, Chien LJ, Lin TL, Yueh YY, Tseng WL, Chang KJ, Wang GR. The epidemiology of Japanese encephalitis on Taiwan during 1966-1997. *Am. J. Trop. Med. Hyg.* 61, 78-84 (1999)

[23] Ayukawa R, Fujimoto H, Ayabe M, Shoji H, Matsui R, Iwata Y, Fukuda H, Ochi K, Noda K, Ono Y, Sakai K, Takehisa Y, Yasui K. An unexpected outbreak of Japanese encephalitis in the Chugoku district of Japan, 2002. *Jpn. J. Infect. Dis.* 57, 63-6 (2002)

[24] Fontenille D Arbovirus transmission cycles in Madagascar. *Arch. Inst. Pasteur. Madagascar.* 55, 311- 7 (1989)

[25] Poidinger M, Hall RA, Mackenzie JS Molecular characterization of the Japanese encephalitis serocomplex of the flavivirus genus. *Virology.* 218, 417-21 (1996)

[26] Daley AJ, Dwyer DE. Emerging viral infections in Australia. *J. Paediatr. Child. Health.* 38, 1-3 (2002)

[27] Mackenzie JS, Johansen CA, Ritchie SA, van den Hurk AF, Hall RA. Japanese encephalitis as an emerging virus: the emergence and spread of Japanese encephalitis virus in Australasia. *Curr. Top. Microbiol. Immunol.* 267, 49-73 (2002)

[28] Pyke AT, Williams DT, Nisbet DJ, van den Hurk AF, Taylor CT, Johansen CA, Macdonald J, Hall RA, Simmons RJ, Mason RJ, Lee JM, Ritchie SA, Smith GA, Mackenzie JS. The appearance of a second genotype of Japanese encephalitis virus in the Australasian region. *Am. J. Trop. Med. Hyg.* 65, 747-53 (2001)

[29] Blumer C, Roche P, Spencer J, Lin M, Milton A, Bunn C, Gidding H, Kaldor J, Kirk M, Hall R, Della-Porta T, Leader R, Wright P; Communicable Diseases Network Australia and subcommittees; Australian Childhood Immunisation Register; Australian Gonococcal Surveillance Programme; Australian Meningococcal Surveillance Programme; Australian Sentinel Practice Research Network; Australian Quarantine Inspection Service; National Centre in HIV Epidemiology and Clinical Research;

National Centre for Immunisation Research and Surveillance of Vaccine Preventable Diseases; National Enteric Pathogens Surveillance Scheme; National Rotavirus Research Centre; Sentinel Chicken Surveillance Programme; National Creutzfeldt-Jakob Disease Registry; World Health Organization Collaborating Centre for Reference and Research on Influenza; Communicable Diseases Control Unit, Australian Capital Territory Department of Health and Community Care, Australian Capital Territory; Communicable Diseases Surveillance and Control Unit, New South Wales Health Department, New South Wales; Centre for Disease Control, Northern Territory Department of Health and Community Services, Northern Territory; Communicable Diseases Unit, Queensland Health, Queensland; Communicable Diseases Control Branch, South Australian Department of Human Services, South Australia; Communicable Diseases Surveillance, Department of Health and Human Services, Tasmania; Communicable Diseases Section, Department of Human Services, Victoria; Communicable Diseases Control Branch, Health Department of Western Australia, Western Australia. Australia's notifiable diseases status, 2001: annual report of the National Notifiable Diseases Surveillance System. *Commun. Dis. Intell.* 27, 1-78 (2003)

[30] Ritchie SA, Pyke AT, Smith GA, Northill JA, Hall RA, van den Hurk AF, Johansen CA, Montgomery BL, Mackenzie JS. Field evaluation of a sentinel mosquito (Diptera: Culicidae) trap system to detect Japanese encephalitis in remote Australia. *J. Med. Entomol.* 40, 249-52 (2003)

[31] Ritchie SA, Rochester W. Wind-blown mosquitoes and introduction of Japanese encephalitis into Australia. *Emerg. Infect. Dis.* 7, 900-3 (2001)

[32] Tiroumourougane SV, Raghava P, Srinivasan S. Japanese viral encephalitis. *Postgrad. Med. J.* 78, 205-15 (2002)

[33] Schwarz TF. Imported vector- and rodent-borne virus infections--an introduction. *Arch. Virol. Suppl.* 11, 3-11 (1996)

[34] Kanojia PC, Geevarghese G. First report on high-degree endophilism in Culex tritaeniorhynchus (Diptera: Culicidae) in an area endemic for Japanese encephalitis. *J. Med. Entomol.* 41, 994-6 (2004)

[35] Arunachalam N, Samuel PP, Hiriyan J, Thenmozhi V, Gajanana A. Japanese encephalitis in Kerala, south India: can Mansonia (Diptera: Culicidae) play a supplemental role in transmission? *J. Med. Entomol.* 41, 456-61 (1994)

[36] Kanojia PC, Shetty PS, Geevarghese G. A long-term study on vector abundance and seasonal prevalence in relation to the occurrence of Japanese encephalitis in Gorakhpur district, Uttar Pradesh. *Indian. J. Med. Res.* 117, 104-10 (2003)

[37] Russell RC, Doggett SL. Japanese encephalitis E. Available at http://medent.usyd.edu.au/fact/japanese%20encephalitis.htm

[38] Mwandawiro C, Boots M, Tuno N, Suwonkerd W, Tsuda Y, Takagi M. Heterogeneity in the host preference of Japanese encephalitis vectors in Chiang Mai, northern Thailand. *Trans. R. Soc. Trop. Med. Hyg.* 94, 238-42 (2000)

[39] Van Den Hurk AF, Johansen CA, Zborowski P, Paru R, Foley PN, Beebe NW, Mackenzie JS, Ritchie SA. Mosquito host-feeding patterns and implications for

Japanese encephalitis virus transmission in northern Australia and Papua New Guinea. *Med. Vet. Entomol.* 17, 403-11 (2003)

[40] Mathur A, Arora KL, Chaturvedi UC. Congenital infection of mice with Japanese encephalitis virus. *Infect. Immun.* 34, 26-9 (1981)

[41] Mathur A, Arora KL, Chaturvedi UC. Transplacental Japanese encephalitis virus (JEV) infection in mice during consecutive pregnancies. *J. Gen. Virol.* 59(Pt 1), 213-7 (1982)

[42] Mathur A, Arora KL, Chaturvedi UC. Immune response to Japanese Encephalitis virus in mother mice and their congenitally infected offspring. *J. Gen. Virol.* 64 (Pt 9), 2027-31 (1983)

[43] Failloux AB, Vazeille-Falcoz M, Mousson L, Rodhain F. Genetic control of vectorial competence in Aedes mosquitoes. *Bull. Soc. Pathol. Exot.* 92, 266-73(1999)

[44] McAda PC, Mason PW, Schmaljohn CS, Dalrymple JM, Mason TL, Fournier MJ. Partial nucleotide sequence of the Japanese encephalitis virus genome. *Virology.* 158, 348-60 (1987)

[45] Nabeshima T, Mori A, Kozaki T, Iwata Y, Hidoh O, Harada S, Kasai S, Severson DW, Kono Y, Tomita T. An amino acid substitution attributable to insecticide-insensitivity of acetylcholinesterase in a Japanese encephalitis vector mosquito, Culex tritaeniorhynchus. *Biochem. Biophys. Res. Commun.* 313, 794-801 (2004)

[46] Miura K, Onodera T, Nishida A, Goto N, Fujisaki Y. A single gene controls resistance to Japanese encephalitis virus in mice. *Arch. Virol.* 112, 261-70 (1990)

[47] Yun SI, Kim SY, Rice CM, Lee YM. Development and application of a reverse genetics system for Japanese encephalitis virus. *J. Virol.* 77, 6450-65 (2003)

[48] Su HL, Liao CL, Lin YL. Japanese encephalitis virus infection initiates endoplasmic reticulum stress and an unfolded protein response. *J. Virol.* 76, 4162-71 (2002)

[49] Lin RJ, Liao CL, Lin E, Lin YL. Blocking of the alpha interferon-induced Jak-Stat signaling pathway by Japanese encephalitis virus infection. *J. Virol.* 78, 9285-94(2004)

[50] Chang YS, Liao CL, Tsao CH, Chen MC, Liu CI, Chen LK, Lin YL. Membrane permeabilization by small hydrophobic nonstructural proteins of Japanese encephalitis virus. *J. Virol.* 73, 6257-64 (1999)

[51] Winter PM, Dung NM, Loan HT, Kneen R, Wills B, Thu le T, House D, White NJ, Farrar JJ, Hart CA, Solomon T. Proinflammatory cytokines and chemokines in humans with Japanese encephalitis. *J. Infect. Dis.* 190, 1618-26 (2004)

[52] Chen CJ, Chen JH, Chen SY, Liao SL, Raung SL. Upregulation of RANTES gene expression in neuroglia by Japanese encephalitis virus infection. *J. Virol.* 78, 12107-19 (2004)

[53] Solomon T, Winter PM. Neurovirulence and host factors in flavivirus encephalitis--evidence from clinical epidemiology. *Arch. Virol. Suppl.* (18), 161-70(2004)

[54] Ravi V, Parida S, Desai A, Chandramuki A, Gourie-Devi M, Grau GE. Correlation of tumor necrosis factor levels in the serum and cerebrospinal fluid with clinical outcome in Japanese encephalitis patients. *J. Med. Virol.* 51, 132-6(1997)

[55] Le DH. Clinical aspects of Japanese B encephalitis in North Vietnam. *Clin. Neurol. Neurosurg.* 88, 189-92 (1986)

[56] Misra UK, Kalita J, Jain SK, Mathur A. Radiological and neurophysiological changes in Japanese encephalitis. *J. Neurol. Neurosurg. Psychiatry.* 57, 1484-7(1994)

[57] Kalita J, Misra UK. EEG in Japanese encephalitis: a clinico-radiological correlation. *Electroencephalogr. Clin. Neurophysiol.* 106, 238-43 (1998)

[58] Misra UK, Kalita J. Seizures in Japanese encephalitis. *J. Neurol. Sci.* 190, 57-60 (2001)

[59] Solomon T, Dung NM, Kneen R, Thao le TT, Gainsborough M, Nisalak A, Day NP, Kirkham FJ, Vaughn DW, Smith S, White NJ. Seizures and raised intracranial pressure in Vietnamese patients with Japanese encephalitis. *Brain.*125, 1084-93(2002)

[60] Solomon T, Dung NM, Kneen R, Thao le TT, Gainsborough M, Nisalak A, Day NP, Kirkham FJ, Vaughn DW, Smith S, White NJ. Seizures and raised intracranial pressure in Vietnamese patients with Japanese encephalitis. *Brain.* 125(Pt 5), 1084-93 (2002)

[61] Misra UK, Kalita J. Anterior horn cells are also involved in Japanese encephalitis. *Acta. Neurol. Scand.* 96, 114-7 (1997)

[62] Solomon T, Kneen R, Dung NM, Khanh VC, Thuy TT, Ha DQ, Day NP, Nisalak A, Vaughn DW, White NJ. Poliomyelitis-like illness due to Japanese encephalitis virus. *Lancet.* 351, 1094-7 (1998)

[63] Misra UK, Kalita J, Srivastava M. Prognosis of Japanese encephalitis: a multivariate analysis. *J. Neurol. Sci.* 161, 143-7 (1998)

[64] Wiwanitkit V. Cerebrospinal fluid examination and interpretation. *Buddhachinaraj. Med. J.* 17, 42 – 52 (2000)

[65] Desai A, Chandramuki A, Gourie-Devi M, Ravi V. Detection of Japanese encephalitis virus antigens in the CSF using monoclonal antibodies. *Clin. Diagn. Virol.* 2, 191-9 (1994)

[66] Buescher EL, Scherer WF. Immunological studies of Japanese encephalitis virus in man. I. Antibody responses following overt infection of man. *J. Immunol.* 83, 582-593 (1959)

[67] Solomon T, Thao LTT, Dung NM, Kneen R, Hung NT, Nisalak A, Vaughn DW, Farrar J, Hien TT, White NJ, Cardosa MJ. Rapid diagnosis of Japanese encephalitis by using an immunoglobulin M dot enzyme immunoassay. *J. Clin. Microbiol.* 36: 2030 - 4 (1998)

[68] Clarke DH, Casals J. Techniques for hemagglutination inhibition with arthropod viruses. *Am. J. Trop. Med. Hyg.* 7:561-573. (1958)

[69] Burke DS, Nisalak A, Ussery MA. Antibody capture immunoassay detection of Japanese encephalitis virus immunoglobulin M and G antibodies in cerebrospinal fluid. *J. Clin. Microbiol.* 16:1034-1042 (1982)

[70] Gadkari DA, Shaikh BH. IgM antibody capture ELISA in the diagnosis of Japanese encephalitis, West Nile and dengue virus infections. *Indian. J. Med. Res.* 80, 613-9 (1984)

[71] Innis BL, Nisalak A, Nimmannitya S, Kusalerdchariya S, Chongswasdi V, Suntayakorn S, Puttisri P, Hoke CH. An enzyme-linked immunosorbent assay to characterize dengue infections where dengue and Japanese encephalitis co-circulate. *Am. J. Trop. Med. Hyg.* 40, 418-427 (1989)

[72] Sun J, Tso S, Chen B. Detection of Japanese encephalitis virus in samples of JE patients by RT-PCR. *Zhonghua. Shi. Yan. He. Lin. Chuang. Bing. Du. Xue. Za. Zhi.* 14, 184-7 (2000)

[73] Huang JL, Lin HT, Wang YM, Weng MH, Ji DD, Kuo MD, Liu HW, Lin CS. Sensitive and specific detection of strains of Japanese encephalitis virus using a one-step TaqMan RT-PCR technique. *J. Med. Virol.* 74, 589-96 (2004)

[74] Yang DK, Kweon CH, Kim BH, Lim SI, Kim SH, Kwon JH, Han HR. TaqMan reverse transcription polymerase chain reaction for the detection of Japanese encephalitis virus. *J. Vet. Sci.* 5, 345-51 (2004)

[75] Miyake M. The pathology of Japanese encephalitis. A review. *Bull. World. Health. Organ.* 30, 153-60 (1964)

[76] Horafuku I. Vitral encephalitis in Japan. Pathology of Japanese encephalitis. *Showa. Igakkai. Zasshi.* 23, 23-5 (1963)

[77] Yamada M, Nakamura K, Yoshii M, Kaku Y. Nonsuppurative encephalitis in piglets after experimental inoculation of Japanese encephalitis flavivirus isolated from pigs. *Vet. Pathol.* 41, 62-7 (2004)

[78] Prakash M, Kumar S, Gupta RK. Diffusion-weighted MR imaging in Japanese encephalitis. *J. Comput. Assist. Tomogr.* 28, 756-61 (2004)

[79] Kalita J, Misra UK. Comparison of CT scan and MRI findings in the diagnosis of Japanese encephalitis. *J. Neurol. Sci.* 174, 3-8 (2000)

[80] Pradhan S, Pandey N, Shashank S, Gupta RK, Mathur A. Parkinsonism due to predominant involvement of substantia nigra in Japanese encephalitis. *Neurology.* 53, 1781-6 (1999)

[81] Johnson RT, Intralawan P, Puapanwatton S. Japanese encephalitis: identification of inflammatory cells in cerebrospinal fluid. *Ann. Neurol.* 20, 691-5 (1986)

[82] Sato Y, Hachiya N, Kuno H, Asoh T, Oizumi K. Cerebrospinal fluid atypical lymphocytes in Japanese encephalitis. *J. Neurol. Sci.* 160, 92-5 (1998)

[83] Kumar R, Mathur A, Singh KB, Sitholey P, Prasad M, Shukla R, Agarwal SP, Arockiasamy J. Clinical sequelae of Japanese encephalitis in children. *Indian. J. Med. Res.* 97, 9-13 (1993)

[84] Shoji H, Watanabe M, Itoh S, Kuwahara H, Hattori F. Japanese encephalitis and parkinsonism. *J. Neurol.* 240, 59-60 (1993)

[85] Goto A. Sequelae of Japanese encephalitis from the viewpoint of neuropsychiatry. *Shinkei. Kenkyu. No. Shimpo.* 11, 329-51 (1967)

[86] Monnet FP. Behavioural disturbances following Japanese B encephalitis. *Eur. Psychiatry.* 18, 269-73 (2003)

[87] Hamano K, Kumada S, Hayashi M, Naito R, Hayashida T, Uchiyama A, Kurata K. Laryngeal dystonia in a case of severe motor and intellectual disabilities due to Japanese encephalitis sequelae. *Brain. Dev.* 26, 335-8 (2004)

[88] Solomon T, Dung NM, Wills B, Kneen R, Gainsborough M, Diet TV, Thuy TT, Loan HT, Khanh VC, Vaughn DW, White NJ, Farrar JJ. Interferon alfa-2a in Japanese encephalitis: a randomised double-blind placebo-controlled trial. *Lancet.* 361, 821-6 (2003)

[89] Saxena SK, Mathur A, Srivastava RC. Inhibition of Japanese encephalitis virus infection by diethyldithiocarbamate is independent of its antioxidant potential. *Antivir. Chem. Chemother.* 14, 91-8 (2003)

[90] Bossi P, Tegnell A, Baka A, van Loock F, Werner A, Hendriks J, Maidhof H, Gouvras G. Bichat patterns for the clinical management of viral encephalitis and bioterrorism-related viral encephalitis. *Euro. Surveil.* 9 (2004)

[91] Wiwanitkit V. Vaccination against mosquito borne viral infections: current status. *Iran. J. Immunol.* 4, 186 – 96 (2007)

[92] Kabilan L. Co ntrol of Japanese encephalitis in India: a reality. *Indian. J. Pediatr.* 71, 707-12 (2004)

[93] Information about Japanese encephalitis vaccine. Available at http://www.metrokc.gov/health/prevcont/encephalitis.htm

[94] Grendel D. Vaccinations for the travellers. *Rev. Prat.* 54, 519-25 (2004)

[95] Lo Re V 3rd, Gluckman SJ. Travel immunizations. *Am. Fam. Physician.* 70, 89-99 (2004)

[96] Plesner AM. Allergic reactions to Japanese encephalitis vaccine. *Immunol. Allergy. Clin. North. Am.* 23, 665-97 (2003)

[97] Plesner A, Ronne T, Wachmann H. Case-control study of allergic reactions to Japanese encephalitis vaccine. *Vaccine.* 18, 1830-6 (2000)

[98] Sakaguchi M, Nakashima K, Takahashi H, Nakayama T, Fujita H, Inouye S. Anaphylaxis to Japanese encephalitis vaccine. *Allergy* 56, 804-5 (2001)

[99] Sakaguchi M, Inouye S. Two patterns of systemic immediate-type reactions to Japanese encephalitis vaccines. *Vaccine.* 16, 68-9 (1998)

[100] Piyasirisilp S, Hemachudha T. Neurological adverse events associated with vaccination. *Curr. Opin. Neurol.* 15, 333-8.(2002)

[101] Kang NG, Oh CW. Gianotti-Crosti syndrome following Japanese encephalitis vaccination. *J. Korean. Med. Sci.* 18, 459-61(2003)

Chapter X

Sandfly Fever

Introduction

Sandfly fever is endemic in the Mediteranian. There are three common groups of sandfly fever virus: Toscana, Naples and Sicily. At present, the widening of epidemiology of sandfly fever to other regions of the world has been mentioned [1]. Sandfly fever is an arbovirus in focus at the present. In this chapter, the brief details of each important sandfly fever virus will be presented and discussed.

Toscana Virus Infection

Toscana virus (*Bunyaviridae* family, *Phlebovirus* genus) is a sandfly fever virus responsible for human neurological infections. Sandfly viruses are transmitted by insect vectors (*Phlebotomus* species) and the infection is present in climatic areas that support the life cycle of the vector [2]. The arthropode-borne Toscana virus is the etiologic agent of meningitis, meningoencephalitis, and encephalitis [2]. Toscana virus was first identified in 1971 from the sandfly *Phlebotomus perniciosus* in central Italy [3]. Many case reports in travelers and clinical research and epidemiologic studies conducted around the Mediterranean region have shown that the virus has a tropism for the central nervous system and is a major cause of meningitis and encephalitis in countries in which it circulates [3]. Considering its epidemiology, in central Italy the virus is the most frequent cause of meningitis from May to October, far exceeding enteroviruses [3]. In the Umbria region of Italy, specific antibodies (IgM and IgG) anti-TOSv were found in 36.6% of aseptic meningitis, in 6.06% of meningoencephalitis and (IgG) in 16% of healthy subjects [4]. In the Tuscany region of Italy, a seroprevalence of Toscana virus of 77.2% among forestry workers was reported [5]. This fact is strictly correlated with the ecological niches specific for the survival of the Toscana virus arthropod vector [5]. Valassina et al. found that there were four variants of the Toscana virus in Tuscany [6]. In Spain, Sanbonmatsu-Gamez et al. reported that the overall seroprevalence rate was 24.9%, significantly increasing with age. They also noted that there is a circulation of at least two different lineages of the virus in the Mediterranean basin, the

Italian lineage and the Spanish lineage [7]. De Ory-Manchon et al. said that the prevalence of the virus in Madrid increased significantly with age [8].

Concerning the clinical manifestation of this viral infection, central nervous system infections are associated with young adults and with a substantially benign clinical course [9]. Navarro et al. studied 17 cases of Toscana virus-induced meningitis [10]. They found that the most common symptoms were headache (holocranial or focal) present in all patients, and moderate fever was observed in 76.5% of the patients with a mean duration of 48 h (range: 18 h–5 days) [10]. All cases were seen between June and October, and predominantly in August [10]. The outcome was favorable in all cases, and the mean time of duration of the disease was seven days (range: 3–10 days) [10]. They conclude that Toscana virus must be taken into account among those agents responsible for lymphocytic meningitis in Spain [10]. Braito et al. performed a similar study in 14 cases of Toscana virus infection in Italy [11]. The study indicates that (1) Toscana virus has been endemic in the Siena province for at least 15 years; (2) the virus is responsible for at least 80% of acute viral infections of the CNS in children throughout the summertime and (3) the clinical signs and symptoms range from aseptic meningitis to meningoencephalitis [11]. In central Italy, acute lymphocytic meningitis and meningoencephalitis due to a Toscana virus occurring throughout the summer are frequently observed [12]. Some atypical cases of neurological infection are also mentioned. Baldelli et al. reported an interesting case of this virus infection presenting with a clinical presentation of stiff neck, deep coma, maculopapular rash, diffuse lymphadenopathy, hepatosplenomegaly, renal involvement, tendency to bleeding, and diffuse intravascular coagulation [13]. Braito et al. proposed that the ecological requirements encompass the conditions in and around the human settlements for phlebotomine sandflies to become peridomestic, thus amplifying the risk of viral infections, which are in fact widespread and frequent in Siena, Italy and its surroundings [12]. In addition to the neurological manifestations, a mild form of Toscana virus infection is also documented. Febrile erythema without meningeal manifestations are reported [14].

Acute lymphocytic meningitis is the clue for diagnosis of this infection. Cerebrospinal fluid examination seems to be a simple tool. For a laboratory diagnostic tool, an enzyme-linked immunosorbent assay (ELISA) based on the recombinant Toscana virus nucleoprotein (rN) was developed in 1999 [15]. Ciufolini et al. found that the sensitivity and specificity of this technique for the detection of virus-specific immunoglobulins G and M in human sera were similar to those of the ELISA, which is based on an antigen extracted from infected mouse brain and that is routinely used for serodiagnosis [15]. In 1999, a recombinant enzyme immunoassay (rEIA) to detect serum immunoglobulin M (IgM) and IgG to Toscana virus (TOSV) was developed by Soldateschi et al. with the aim of establishing a simple and easily available assay for diagnosing acute or previous infections [16]. According to this work, the overall sensitivity and specificity of rEIA were both 100% for IgM detection and 100 and 96.6%, respectively, for IgG detection [16]. Soldateschi et al. proposed that rEIA appeared to be a simple and reliable laboratory test for the diagnosis of acute Toscana infection and for the assessment of immune status [16]. The molecular diagnostic technique for this infection has also been developed. In 2002, Valassina et al. developed a fast duplex one-step RT-PCR for rapid differential diagnosis of entero- or Toscana virus meningitis [17]. They proposed that the multiplex one-step RT-nPCR protocol allowed for the detection of enterovirus and

Toscana virus RNA in a single sample, by using, at the same time, a very small clinical sample volume [17]. In 2007, Ruiz et al. described a new reverse transcription, real-time PCR assay for detection of both Toscana virus genotypes [18]. According to this work, the sensitivity of the assay was 0.0158 TICD(50) per reaction of Toscana virus, equivalent to seven copies of cDNA. No other phleboviruses or RNA viruses were amplified by this specific real-time PCR [18]. Ruiz et al. proposed that the assay seemed to be sensitive, reliable and easy to be applied in the diagnosis of autochthonous or imported suspected cases of Toscana virus infection [18].

Similar to general viral meningitis disease, specific treatment for Toscana virus infection is not available. Although an antiviral drug, ribavirin, is used, the efficacy is not favorable. For prevention, vector control is recommended. No vaccine is available.

Naples Virus Infection

Sandfly fever Naples viruses were first isolated from sick persons during World War II [19]. This infection is common in Southern Italy. Antibody prevalence rate of 57% is reported in Cyprus [20]. In addition to the Mediteranian, Naples virus infection can also be seen in other areas of the world. Naples virus activity is reported in Iran [21], Sudan [22] and Israel [23]. Considering the clinical manifestations, the same manifestations as those of Toscana virus infection are documented. Concerning laboratory abnormalities, differential blood count can show a lymphocytopenia, and cerebrospinal fluid can show lymphocytic profile [24]. Other abnormal laboratory findings include an elevated blood sedimentation rate and a slightly increased C-reactive protein value [24].

Sicily Virus Infection

Similar to Naples virus, sandfly fever Sicily viruses were first isolated from sick persons during World War II [19]. The endemic areas of this infection are the two main islands, Sicily and Sardinia [20]. Considering the clinical manifestations, the same manifestations as those of Toscana virus infection have been documented.

References

[1] Sanchez-Seco MP, Navarro JM. Infections due to Toscana virus, West Nile virus, and other arboviruses of interest in Europe. *Enferm. Infecc. Microbiol. Clin.* 23, 560-8 (2005)

[2] Valassina M, Cusi MG, Valensin PE. A Mediterranean arbovirus: the Toscana virus. *J. Neurovirol.* 9, 577-83 (2003)

[3] Charrel RN, Gallian P, Navarro-Mari JM, Nicoletti L, Papa A, Sanchez-Seco MP, Tenorio A, de Lamballerie X. Emergence of Toscana virus in Europe. *Emerg. Infect. Dis.* 11, 1657-63 (2005)

[4] Francisci D, Papili R, Camanni G, Morosi S, Ferracchiato N, Valente M, Ciufolini MG, Baldelli F. Evidence of Toscana virus circulation in Umbria: first report. *Eur. J. Epidemiol.* 18, 457-9 (2003)

[5] Sanbonmatsu-Gamez S, Perez-Ruiz M, Collao X, Sanchez-Seco MP, Morillas-Marquez F, de la Rosa-Fraile M, Navarro-Mari JM, Tenorio A. Toscana virus in Spain. *Emerg. Infect. Dis.* 11, 1701-7 (2005)

[6] Valassina M, Valentini M, Pugliese A, Valensin PE, Cusi MG. Serological survey of Toscana virus infections in a high-risk population in Italy. *Clin. Diagn. Lab. Immunol.* 10, 483-4 (2003)

[7] Valassina M, Cuppone AM, Bianchi S, Santini L, Cusi MG. Evidence of Toscana virus variants circulating in Tuscany, Italy, during the summers of 1995 to 1997. *J. Clin. Microbiol.* 36, 2103-4 (1998)

[8] de Ory-Manchon F, Sanz-Moreno JC, Aranguez-Ruiz E, Ramirez-Fernandez R. Age-dependent seroprevalence of Toscana virus in the Community of Madrid: 1993-1994 and 1999-2000. *Enferm. Infecc. Microbiol. Clin.* 25, 187 (2007)

[9] Di Nicuolo G, Pagliano P, Battisti S, Starace M, Mininni V, Attanasio V, Faella FS. Toscana virus central nervous system infections in southern Italy. *J. Clin. Microbiol.* 43, 6186-8 (2005)

[10] Navarro JM, Fernandez-Roldan C, Perez-Ruiz M, Sanbonmatsu S, de la Rosa M, Sanchez-Seco MP. Meningitis by Toscana virus in Spain: description of 17 cases. *Med. Clin. (Barc).* 122, 420-2 (2004)

[11] Braito A, Corbisiero R, Corradini S, Fiorentini C, Ciufolini MG. Toscana virus infections of the central nervous system in children: a report of 14 cases. *J. Pediatr.* 132, 144-8 (1998)

[12] Braito A, Corbisiero R, Corradini S, Marchi B, Sancasciani N, Fiorentini C, Ciufolini MG. Evidence of Toscana virus infections without central nervous system involvement: a serological study. *Eur. J. Epidemiol.* 13, 761-4 (1997)

[13] Baldelli F, Ciufolini MG, Francisci D, Marchi A, Venturi G, Fiorentini C, Luchetta ML, Bruto L, Pauluzzi S. Unusual presentation of life-threatening Toscana virus meningoencephalitis. *Clin. Infect. Dis.* 38, 515-20 (2004)

[14] Portolani M, Sabbatini AM, Beretti F, Gennari W, Tamassia MG, Pecorari M. Symptomatic infections by toscana virus in the Modena province in the triennium 1999-2001. *New. Microbiol.* 25, 485-8 (2002)

[15] Ciufolini MG, Fiorentini C, di Bonito P, Mochi S, Giorgi C. Detection of Toscana virus-specific immunoglobulins G and M by an enzyme-linked immunosorbent assay based on recombinant viral nucleoprotein. *J. Clin. Microbiol.* 37, 2010-2 (1999)

[16] Soldateschi D, dal Maso GM, Valassina M, Santini L, Bianchi S, Cusi MG. Laboratory diagnosis of Toscana virus infection by enzyme immunoassay with recombinant viral nucleoprotein. *J. Clin. Microbiol.* 37, 649-52 (1999)

[17] Valassina M, Valentini M, Valensin PE, Cusi MG. Fast duplex one-step RT-PCR for rapid differential diagnosis of entero- or toscana virus meningitis. *Diagn. Microbiol Infect. Dis.* 43, 201-5 (2002)

[18] Ruiz M, Collao X, Navarro-Mari JM, Tenorio A. Reversetranscription, real-time PCR assay for detection of Toscana virus. *J. Clin. Virol.* 39, 276-81 (2007)

[19] Verani P, Nicoletti L, Ciufolini MG, Balducci M. Viruses transmitted by sandflies in Italy. *Parassitologia.* 33 Suppl, 513-8 (1991)

[20] Eitrem R, Stylianou M, Niklasson B. High prevalence rates of antibody to three sandfly fever viruses (Sicilian, Naples, and Toscana) among Cypriots. *Epidemiol. Infect.* 107, 685-91 (1991)

[21] Saidi S, Tesh R, Javadian E, Sahabi Z, Nadim A. Studies on the epidemiology of sandfly fever in Iran. II. The prevalence of human and animal infection with five phlebotomus fever virus serotypes in Isfahan province. *Am. J. Trop. Med. Hyg.* 26, 288-93 (1977)

[22] Watts DM, el-Tigani A, Botros BA, Salib AW, Olson JG, McCarthy M, Ksiazek TG. Arthropod-borne viral infections associated with a fever outbreak in the northern province of Sudan. *J. Trop. Med. Hyg.* 97, 228-30 (1994)

[23] Cohen D, Zaide Y, Karasenty E, Schwarz M, LeDuc JW, Slepon R, Ksiazek TG, Shemer J, Green MS. Prevalence of antibodies to West Nile fever, sandfly fever Sicilian, and sandfly fever Naples viruses in healthy adults in Israel. *Public. Health. Rev.* 27, 217-30 (1999)

[24] Imirzalioglu C, Schaller M, Bretzel RG. Sandfly fever Naples virus (serotype Toscana) infection with meningeal involvement after a vacation in Italy. *Dtsch. Med. Wochenschr.* 131, 2838-40 (2006)

[25] Maroli M, Bigliocchi F, Khoury C. Sandflies in Italy: observations on their distribution and methods for control. *Parassitologia.* 36, 251-64 (1994)

Chapter XI

Minor Arbovirus Hemorrhagic Fever

Chikungunya Infection

A. Introduction

Chikungunya infection is a viral infection causing hemorrhagic fever similar to dengue virus infection. Chikungunya virus is classified as an arbovirus (group A).

It is a virus in the *Togaviridae* family [1]. Chikungunya fever is a disease transmitted to human beings by *Aedes* genus mosquitoes [1]. Chikungunya virus is highly infective. An incubation period of 3–12 days is noted [2-3]. With regard to the clinical manifestations, sudden severe headache, chills, fever, joint pain and muscle pain are the most common symptoms [3]. Children can show neurological symptoms [3]. Hemorrhagic fever is a serious complication of this infection. The hemorrhage is rare and can resolve in three to five days [3]. Detection of antigens or antibodies of the agent in blood is the main diagnosis for this infection. An IgM ELISA is necessary to distinguish the illness from dengue fever [3]. The application of molecular diagnosis to Chikungunya virus infection of is also proposed [3]. The acute hemorrhagic fever caused by Chikungunya infection can be treated with protocols similar to dengue fever (Table 1).

Table 1. Comparison on hemorrhagic fever caused by dengue and Chikungunya infections

Clinical parameter	Dengue	Chikungunya
Pathogen	Dengue virus	Chikungunya virus
Vector	*Aedes aegypti*	*Aedes aegypti*
Thrombocytopenia	More common	Less common
Leukocytopenia	Less common	More common
Tourniquet test	Positive	Positive
Induction of shock	More common	Less common
Treatment	Supportive	Supportive

Wiwanikit V, 2005.

B. Vector and Epidemiology

As previously mentioned, Chikungunya can share a common vector with dengue virus. *Aedes* mosquitoes seem to be the main vector for this infection. The disease typically consists of an acute illness characterised by fever, rash, and incapacitating arthralgia. The word chikungunya, used for both the virus and the disease, means "to walk bent over" in some east African languages, and refers to the effect of the joint pain that characterizes this dengue-like infection [4]. Chikungunya is a specifically tropical disease, but it is geographically restricted and outbreaks are relatively uncommon [4]. *Aedes aegypti* and *Aedes albopictus* are the two main mosquito vectors [5]. Similar to dengue, vector abundance is the main determinant factor for Chikungunya infection. Emergence of this infection is believed to strongly relate to distribution of mosquitoes [6]. A recent example is the outbreak of Chikungunya on the Indian Ocean island of Reunion [7]. Pialoux et al. said that plausible explanations for the new emergence of Chikungunya infection include increased tourism, Chikungunya virus introduction into a naïve population, and viral mutation.

According to the study of Powers et al., phylogenetic trees corroborated historical evidence that Chikungunya virus originated in Africa and subsequently was introduced into Asia [8]. Within the eastern Africa and southern Africa/Asia lineage, Asian strains grouped together in a genotype distinct from the African groups [8]. These different geographical genotypes exhibit differences in their transmission cycles: in Asia, the virus appears to be maintained in an urban cycle with *Aedes aegypti* mosquito vectors [8], while Chikungunya virus transmission in Africa involves a sylvatic cycle, primarily with *Aedes furcifer* and *Aedes africanus* mosquitoes [8-9]. A sylvatic cycle type was well demonstrated in a recent study by Diallo et al. in Senegal [9]. With no vaccine or antiviral medication available, prevention and control depend on surveillance, early identification of outbreaks, and vector control [5].

C. Pathogenesis

The pathogenesis of Chikungunya infection is similar to dengue fever. A hemorrhagic episode is believed to be an immunological mimicking process. Arthritis seems to be due to the same process. For the outbreak, the molecular shift is also important. The unique molecular features of the analyzed Indian Ocean isolates of chikungunya virus demonstrate their high evolutionary potential and suggest possible clues for understanding the atypical magnitude and virulence of the recent outbreak in Indian Ocean territories [10-11].

D. Clinical Manifestation and Diagnosis

Clinical manifestation of Chikungunya virus infection is similar to that of dengue infection. Important presentations are characterized by fever, eruptions and invalidating arthralgia [12-13]. Although viral diagnostics (culture, serological tests and polymerase chain reaction tests) can be used to confirm the infection, these tests are not accessible during outbreaks to the majority of the population in the poor underdeveloped endemic areas [14]. Chikungunya fever must be a suspected in travelers who develop fever and arthritis after traveling to areas affected by an ongoing epidemic [15]. Related arthritis mainly affects smaller joints and often persists for extended periods [15]. Serological testing may have negative results during the first week of the disease; diagnosis using polymerase chain reaction appears to be more reliable during this time [15].

E. Treatment

Similar to dengue infection, there is no specific treatment for Chikunganya infection. Symptomatic treatment, especially for fluid replacement therapy, is needed. There are some trials using chloroquine for treatment of chronic arthritis in Chikunganya infection [16]. Basically, more than 12% of patients who contract Chikungunya virus infection develop chronic joint symptoms [16]. These symptoms respond only partially to non-steroidal anti-inflammatory drugs [16]. However, there is no clear-cut report that chloroquine is effective.

F. Prevention

Vector control is still the best method, similar to dengue infection. Vaccine for this infection is available. Formalin-inactivated Chikungunya vaccines have been developed for decades [17-18]. Is was also noted that Chikungunya virus vaccines prepared by Tween 80 and ether inactivation of virus grown in green monkey kidney cell cultures were shown to be immunogenic, comparable with Formalin-inactivated vaccines [19]. Recently, an attenuated Chikungunya virus clone was developed for production of a live vaccine for human use [20]. Because of the low viremias produced in inoculated humans, it is unlikely that mosquitoes would become infected by feeding on a person inoculated with the live attenuated vaccine [21]. It was reported that this new vaccine was safe, produced well-tolerated side effects, and was highly immunogenic [22]. Although the vaccine was transmitted by mosquitoes after intrathoracic inoculation, there was no evidence of reversion to a virulent phenotype [21].

Crimean-Congo Hemorrhagic Fever

Crimean-Congo hemorrhagic fever (CCHF) is another arboviral hemorrhagic fever. It is a tick-borne disease caused by the arbovirus Crimean-Congo hemorrhagic fever virus (CCHFV), which is a member of the *Nairovirus* genus (family *Bunyaviridae*) [23]. CCHF was first recognized during a large outbreak among agricultural workers in the mid-1940s in the Crimean peninsula [23]. The disease now occurs sporadically throughout much of Africa, Asia, and Europe and results in an approximately 30% fatality rate [23]. Numerous genera of ixodid ticks serve both as vector and reservoir for CCHFV [23]. Exposure to ticks, particularly those in the genus *Hyalomma*, or direct contact with virus-infected animals or people, are considered the major risk factors [24].

There are some interesting epidemiological reports on CCHF. Izadi et al. performed an interesting study to assess the seroprevalence of CCHF virus infection within the Zahedan and Zabol districts of the Sistan-va-Baluchestan province in Iran [25]. In this work, 300 subjects were sampled from the general population [25] and the point estimate of the seroprevalence was 0.024 [25]. Izadi et al. reported that CCHF in Iran did not differ substantially from other parts of the world [26]. Jabbari et al. said that humans were usually infected with CCHF virus through a tick bite or close contact with viral contaminated tissues or with blood of domestic animals or of infected patients [27]. Even though tick bite is one of the most important risk factors for CCHF, it cannot explain all cases and there are other important risk factors such as high-risk occupations and having contact with livestock [26]. Smirnova reported that the circulation of CCHF in the Stavropol territory of Russia in 14 regions out of 24 expected was established [28]. Smirnova said that an essential factor of the exacerbation of the epidemic situation was a rise in the number of *Hyalomma marginatum* ticks, the main vector of the causative agent of CCHF in the south of Russia [28]. Rodriguez et al. performed a study on molecular investigation of a multisource outbreak of CCHF in the United Arab Emirates [29]. Within this lineage, sequences from the UAE patients were identical or closely related to those from three *Hyalomma* spp. ticks obtained from livestock recently imported from Somalia [29]. Another sequence from a UAE patient was more closely related to a CCHF virus from Nigeria [29]. A cross-sectional seroprevalence survey in Senegal was performed by Chapman et al. [30]. According to this work, human infection of CCHF occurred more frequently or with less mortality in the region studied than has been found elsewhere in Africa; however, the rate of seroconversion-associated illness is undetermined. Hyalomma ticks appear to be the primary transmission mode [30]. Williams et al. studied the seroprevalence of CCHF in Oman [31]. In this work, butchers were more likely to have CCHF antibody than persons in other job categories [31]. The presence of clinical disease and the serological results for animals and humans and infected *Hyalomma* ticks provide ample evidence of the presence of CCHF virus in yet another country in the Arabian Peninsula [31].

Recent advances in molecular and biochemical analyses of CCHF virus revealed that the virus encodes larger proteins compared to other genera of *Bunyaviridae* and the processing of viral proteins are complicated [32]. Recent studies also showed that the CCHF viruses are relatively divergent in their genome sequence and the viruses are grouped in seven different clades [32]. These are completely conserved among the predicted polyprotein sequences of all the CCHF virus strains and closely resemble the tetrapeptides that represent the major cleavage recognition sites present in the glycoprotein precursors of arenaviruses, such as Lassa fever virus and Pichinde virus [33]. These results strongly suggest that CCHF viruses (and other members of the genus *Nairovirus*) likely utilize the subtilase SKI-1/S1P-like cellular proteases for the major glycoprotein precursor cleavage events, as has recently been demonstrated for the arenaviruses [33]. Hewson et al. studied the phylogenetic patter of three datasets of sequences from the small genomic RNA segment available from a range of strains of CCHF viruses and found that CCHF virus could be divided into seven subtypes [34]. Superimposed on this pattern are links between distant geographic locations, pointing to the existence of a global reservoir of CCHF virus [34]. In some cases these links may originate from trade in livestock, and long-distance carriage of virus or infected ticks during bird migration [34]. Deyde et al. noted that discrepancies among the virus S, M, and L phylogenetic tree topologies documented multiple RNA segment reassortment events [35]. They suggested genetic recombination also occurred and the genomic plasticity of CCHF virus is surprisingly high for an arthropod-borne virus [35].

After a short incubation period, CCHF is characterized by a sudden onset of high fever, chills, severe headache, dizziness, back, and abdominal pains. Additional symptoms can include nausea, vomiting, diarrhea, and neuropsychiatric and cardiovascular changes [23]. In addition to previously reported symptoms and signs, Karti et al. report hemophagocytosis in 50% of our patients, which is the first report of this clinical phenomenon associated with CCHF [36]. Also, an unusual cause of acute abdominal pain simulating acute appendicitis was also presented [37]. In this case, the patient was admitted with complaints of fever, malaise, headache, nausea, vomiting, diarrhea, and severe bleeding [37]. Based on the clinical and epidemiological findings, a diagnosis of CCHF virus infection was suspected, and ribavirin therapy was started [37]. In severe cases, hemorrhagic manifestations, ranging from petechiae to large areas of ecchymosis, developed [24]. Schwarz et al. studied the clinical features of CHHF cases in the United Arab Emirates [38]. In this series, about 70% of the cases were fatal [38]. Symptoms started 3.5 days before hospitalization. On admission, 81.8% of patients had high fever, 45.5% were vomiting, 63.6% had diarrhea, 45.5% had haemorrhagic signs, and 18.2% had throat pain [38]. A hospital outbreak of haemorrhagic fever took place in Dubai in November, 1979 [39]. The index case died in the casualty department shortly after admission [39]. In this case series, there were five secondary cases among hospital staff, two of whom died [39].

Baskerville et al. studied the histopathology of CCHF and reported that histopathological changes included extensive cellular necrosis and hemorrhage in the liver, necrosis and lymphoid depletion in the spleen, congestion and edema formation in the lungs, and hemorrhage in a number of other organs [40]. For diagnosis of infection, serological testing is widely used. In diagnosis, enzyme-linked immunoassays are widely used [41]. Early diagnosis is critical for patient therapy and prevention of potential nosocomial infections [41]. The new molecular biology technique, RT-PCR, allows rapid detection of genomic CCHF viral RNA in clinical specimens and study of the molecular epidemiology of this infection [42]. However, this test is expensive and might not be suitable for long distance in underdeveloped endemic areas.

For treatment, supportive treatment is the core. Careful maintenance of fluid and electrolyte balance, circulatory volume, and blood pressure are recommended [43-45]. Since an effective vaccine and a specific antiviral therapy has not yet been found, the high mortality rate may reach 10–60% [43]. The CCHF virus is susceptible to ribavirin in vitro but there is no controlled study evaluating oral versus intravenous ribavirin in treating Crimean-Congo hemorrhagic fever patients, and few studies have evaluated oral ribavirin [45]. Impaired consciousness and splenomegaly are independent predictors of a fatal outcome [44]. The increasing worldwide medical awareness, the enormous interest of the media in hemorrhagic fever diseases, and their potential to be used as a bioweapon have greatly spurred research on this important virus, as evidenced by many new developments, including the development of a reverse genetics system which should greatly enhance future research on this virus [46].

Alkhumra Virus Infection

This infection is not a well-known viral infection. This new flavivirus was originally isolated in 1995 from six patients with dengue-like hemorrhagic fever from the Alkhumra district, south of Jeddah, Saudi Arabia. Considering the clinical manifestations of this disease, Madani reported that acute febrile flu-like illness with hepatitis (100%), hemorrhagic manifestations (55%), and encephalitis (20%) were the main clinical features [47]. Madani noted that the case fatality was 25% [47]. They proposed that the disease seemed to be transmitted from sheep or goats to humans by mosquito bites or direct contact with these animals [48]. In 2001, Charrel et al. reported the complete coding sequence of Alkhumra virus, which was determined to be 10,248 nucleotides (nt) long, and to encode a single 3,416 amino acid polyprotein [48]. Independent analyses of the complete polyprotein and the envelope protein provided genetic and phylogenetic evidence that Alkhumra virus belongs to the tick-borne flavivirus group, within which it is most closely related to Kyasanur Forest disease virus [48]. Pauci-symptomatic or asymptomatic cases are likely, but epidemiologic data are currently unavailable [49]. Until the present, the role of arthropods such as ticks and mosquitoes, and animals such as sheep, goats, and rodents in the transmission and maintenance of the virus remains to be elucidated. However, current evidence suggests that transmission to humans can occur either transcutaneously either by contamination of a skin wound with the blood of an infected vertebrate or the bites of an infected tick or orally by drinking unpasteurized contaminated milk [49].

In 2007, one *Ornithodoros savignyi* tick from Saudi Arabia was found to contain this virus RNA [50]. This is the first direct evidence that Alkhumra virus is a tick-borne flavivirus and confirms the association between human Alkhumra virus cases and tick bite history [50]. Charrel said that this infection must be considered as a new emerging tick-borne arbovirus infection [50-51]. Since viral diagnosis and vaccine development may be hindered by genetic diversity, Charrel et al. found that the diversity observed within the studied Alkhumra virus strains in Saudi Arabia reflected a 4- to 72-year period of evolution [52].

Malpais Spring Virus Infection

This infection is also another uncommon viral infection. In 1985, two virus isolates, one each from *A. campestris* and *Psorophora signipennis* mosquitoes, were collected in south central New Mexico in August 1985 [53]. The name Malpais Spring virus is proposed for this newly-recognized vesiculovirus. A serologic survey indicated that Malpais Spring virus infects indigenous (mule deer and pronghorn) and exotic (gemsbok) ungulates at and near the sites where the mosquitoes, from which the virus strains were isolated, were collected [53]. Antibody prevalence in wild animals indicates that the pronghorn and gemsbok may play roles as hosts for Malpais Spring epizootic hemorrhagic disease in New Jersey [53]. For human infection, to the present, there has been no report of this viral infection.

Omsk Hemorrhagic Fever Virus Infection

Omsk hemorrhagic fever virus infection is a new arboviral infection. The etiological agent is a member of flavivirus, similar to dengue virus. First it was classified as a tick-borne hemorrhagic flavivirus [54]. Presently, it is suspected that this infection can also be a mosquito-transmitted disease. Recently, Volk et al. solved the NMR solution structure of domain III from the Omsk hemorrhagic fever virus envelope protein and reported the first sequencing of the Guriev strain of this virus [55]. Important structural differences exist between Omsk hemorrhagic fever virus and mosquito-borne flaviviruses, such as West Nile virus [55]. This finding can lead to the possible assumption that this infection is tick-borne rather than mosquito-borne.

Bivens Arm Virus Infection

During field studies in 1981 on the transmission of bluetongue viruses in ruminants in Florida, a virus was isolated from *Culicoides insignis* midges (a tiny fly-like insect) collected near water buffalo (*Bubalus bubalis*) recently imported from Trinidad [56]. The virus is classified as a member of the Tibrogargan group, members of which have hitherto been found only in Australasia [57]. They are considered to be transmitted by the *Culicoides* species [57]. Electron microscopy showed that this isolate, for which the name Bivens Arm virus is proposed, has rhabdovirus morphology [56]. Serologic comparisons were made with recognized rhabdoviruses from terrestrial vertebrates and hematophagous arthropods [56]. Up to the present, there has been no report of this viral infection in humans.

Blue Tongue Virus Infection

Blue tongue virus infection is another important veterinarian arbovirus infection. Bluetongue virus is transmitted by midges, and can cause serious disease in sheep. Both virus neutralizing antibodies and cytotoxic T lymphocytes have been shown to have a role in protective immunity [58]. Recently, Ibaraki disease, an epizootic disease of cattle in Japan resembling bluetongue, is characterized by fever and lesions affecting the mucous membranes, skin, musculature and vascular system [59]. Degeneration of striated muscular tissue is observed in the esophagus, larynx, pharynx, tongue and skeletal muscles. Edema and haemorrhage are marked in the mouth, lips, abomasum, around the coronets, etc. [59].

Kyasanur Forest Disease

Kyasanur forest disease (KFD) was first recognised as a febrile illness in the Shimoga district of Karnataka state in India [60]. The causative agent, KFD virus (KFDV), is a highly pathogenic member in the family *Flaviviridae*, producing a haemorrhagic disease in infected human beings. KFD is a zoonotic disease and has so far been localised only in a southern part of India [60]. The disease is classified as a new tick-borne infection. The early clinical description of the disease includes severe cases with hemorrhagic manifestations, including intermittent epistaxis, hematemesis, melena, and frank blood in the stools [61]. Pathological and hematological investigations emphasize many similarities with Omsk hemorrhagic fever [61]. Recently, a formalin inactivated KFD virus tissue culture vaccine was produced by the health department of the State Government of Karnataka [62]. Dandawate et al. reported that the vaccine has a highly significant protective effect [62]. Of interest, in addition to human infections, epizootic disease in monkeys has also been widely mentioned [63-64].

References

[1] Diallo M, Thonnon J, Traore-Lamizana M, Fontenille D. Vectors of Chikungunya virus in Senegal: current data and transmission cycles. *Am. J. Trop. Med. Hyg.* 60, 281-6 (1999)

[2] Chikungunya infection. Available at http://www.cbwinfo.com/Biological/Pathogens/CHIK.html

[3] Andrei G, De Clercq E. Molecular approaches for the treatment of hemorrhagic fever virus infections. *Antiviral. Res.* 22, 45-75 (1993)

[4] Pialoux G, Gauzere BA, Jaureguiberry S, Strobel M. Chikungunya, an epidemic arbovirosis. *Lancet. Infect. Dis.* 7, 319-27 (2007)

[5] Sam IC, AbuBakar S. Chikungunya virus infection. *Med. J. Malaysia.* 61, 264-9 (2006)

[6] Pages F, Corbel V, Paupy C. Aedes albopictus as an epidemic vector of chikungunya virus: another emerging problem? *Lancet. Infect. Dis.* 6, 463-4 (2006)

[7] Pages F, Corbel V, Paupy C. Aedes albopictus: chronical of a spreading vector. *Med. Trop.* (Mars). 66, 226-8 (2006)

[8] Powers AM, Brault AC, Tesh RB, Weaver SC. Re-emergence of Chikungunya and O'nyong-nyong viruses: evidence for distinct geographical lineages and distant evolutionary relationships. *J. Gen. Virol.* (Pt 2), 471-9 (2000)

[9] Diallo M, Thonnon J, Traore-Lamizana M, Fontenille D. Vectors of Chikungunya virus in Senegal: current data and transmission cycles. *Am. J. Trop. Med. Hyg.* 60, 281-6 (1999)

[10] Schuffenecker I, Iteman I, Michault A, Murri S, Frangeul L, Vaney MC, Lavenir R, Pardigon N, Reynes JM, Pettinelli F, Biscornet L, Diancourt L, Michel S, Duquerroy S, Guigon G, Frenkiel MP, Brehin AC, Cubito N, Despres P, Kunst F, Rey FA, Zeller H, Brisse S. Genome microevolution of chikungunya viruses causing the Indian Ocean outbreak. *PLoS. Med.* 3, e263 (2006)

[11] Arankalle VA, Shrivastava S, Cherian S, Gunjikar RS, Walimbe AM, Jadhav SM, Sudeep AB, Mishra AC. Genetic divergence of Chikungunya viruses in India (1963-2006) with special reference to the 2005-2006 explosive epidemic. *J. Gen. Virol.* 88(Pt 7), 1967-76 (2007)

[12] Nakoune E, Finance C, Le Faou A, Rihn B. The Chikungunya virus. *Ann. Biol. Clin. (Paris).* 65, 349-56 (2007)

[13] Mohan A. Chikungunya fever: clinical manifestations and management. *Indian. J. Med. Res.* 124, 471-4 (2006)

[14] Kalantri SP, Joshi R, Riley LW. Chikungunya epidemic: an Indian perspective. *Natl. Med. J. India.* 19, 315-22 (2006)

[15] Taubitz W, Cramer JP, Kapaun A, Pfeffer M, Drosten C, Dobler G, Burchard GD, Loscher T. Chikungunya fever in travelers: clinical presentation and course. *Clin. Infect. Dis.* 45, e1-4 (2007)

[16] Brighton SW. Chloroquine phosphate treatment of chronic Chikungunya arthritis. An open pilot study. *S. Afr. Med. J.* 66, 217-8 (1984)

[17] Eckels KH, Harrison VR, Hetrick FM. Chikungunya virus vaccine prepared by Tween-ether extraction. *Appl. Microbiol.* 19, 321-5 (1970)

[18] Harrison VR, Eckels KH, Bartelloni PJ, Hampton C. Production and evaluation of a formalin-killed Chikungunya vaccine. *J. Immunol.* 107, 643-7 (1971)

[19] White A, Berman S, Lowenthal JP. Comparative immunogenicities of Chikungunya vaccines propagated in monkey kidney monolayers and chick embryo suspension cultures. *Appl. Microbiol.* 23, 951-2 (1972)

[20] Levitt NH, Ramsburg HH, Hasty SE, Repik PM, Cole FE Jr, Lupton HW. Development of an attenuated strain of chikungunya virus for use in vaccine production. *Vaccine.* 4, 157-62 (1986)

[21] Turell MJ, Malinoski FJ. Limited potential for mosquito transmission of a live, attenuated chikungunya virus vaccine. *Am. J. Trop. Med. Hyg.* 47, 98-103 (1992)

[22] Edelman R, Tacket CO, Wasserman SS, Bodison SA, Perry JG, Mangiafico JA. Phase II safety and immunogenicity study of live chikungunya virus vaccine TSI-GSD-218. *Am. J. Trop. Med. Hyg.* 62, 681-5 (2000)

[23] Whitehouse CA. Crimean-Congo hemorrhagic fever. *Antiviral. Res.* 64, 145-60 (2004)

[24] Flick R, Whitehouse CA. Crimean-Congo hemorrhagic fever virus. *Curr. Mol. Med.* 5, 753-60 (2005)

[25] Izadi S, Holakouie-Naieni K, Majdzadeh SR, Chinikar S, Nadim A, Rakhshani F, Hooshmand B. Seroprevalence of Crimean-Congo hemorrhagic fever in Sistan-va-Baluchestan province of Iran. *Jpn. J. Infect. Dis.* 59, 326-8 (2006)

[26] Izadi S, Naieni KH, Madjdzadeh SR, Nadim A. Crimean-Congo hemorrhagic fever in Sistan and Baluchestan Province of Iran, a case-control study on epidemiological characteristics. *Int. J. Infect. Dis.* 8, 299-306 (2004)

[27] Jabbari A, Besharat S, Abbasi A, Moradi A, Kalavi K. Crimean-Congo hemorrhagic fever: case series from a medical center in Golestan province, Northeast of Iran (2004). *Indian. J. Med. Sci.* 60, 327-9 (2006)

[28] Smirnova SE. Circulation of Crimean-Congo hemorrhagic fever virus in the Stavropol territory in the seasons of 1999-2000. *Zh. Mikrobiol. Epidemiol. Immunobiol.* 3, 49-53 (2005)

[29] Rodriguez LL, Maupin GO, Ksiazek TG, Rollin PE, Khan AS, Schwarz TF, Lofts RS, Smith JF, Noor AM, Peters CJ, Nichol ST. Molecular investigation of a multisource outbreak of Crimean-Congo hemorrhagic fever in the United Arab Emirates. *Am. J. Trop. Med. Hyg.* 57, 512-8 (1997)

[30] Chapman LE, Wilson ML, Hall DB, LeGuenno B, Dykstra EA, Ba K, Fisher-Hoch SP. Risk factors for Crimean-Congo hemorrhagic fever in rural northern Senegal. *J. Infect. Dis.* 164, 686-92 (1991)

[31] Williams RJ, Al-Busaidy S, Mehta FR, Maupin GO, Wagoner KD, Al-Awaidy S, Suleiman AJ, Khan AS, Peters CJ, Ksiazek TG. Crimean-congo haemorrhagic fever: a seroepidemiological and tick survey in the Sultanate of Oman. *Trop. Med. Int. Health.* 5,99 – 106 (2000)

[32] Morikawa S, Saijo M, Kurane I. Recent progress in molecular biology of Crimean-Congo hemorrhagic fever. *Comp. Immunol. Microbiol. Infect. Dis.* (2007) Aug 9; [Epub ahead of print]

[33] Sanchez AJ, Vincent MJ, Nichol ST. Characterization of the glycoproteins of Crimean-Congo hemorrhagic fever virus. *J. Virol.* 76, 7263-75 (2002)

[34] Hewson R, Chamberlain J, Mioulet V, Lloyd G, Jamil B, Hasan R, Gmyl A, Gmyl L, Smirnova SE, Lukashev A, Karganova G, Clegg C. Crimean-Congo haemorrhagic fever virus: sequence analysis of the small RNA segments from a collection of viruses world wide. *Virus. Res.* 102, 185-9 (2004)

[35] Deyde VM, Khristova ML, Rollin PE, Ksiazek TG, Nichol ST. Crimean-Congo hemorrhagic fever virus genomics and global diversity. *J. Virol.* 80, 8834-42 (2006)

[36] Karti SS, Odabasi Z, Korten V, Yilmaz M, Sonmez M, Caylan R, Akdogan E, Eren N, Koksal I, Ovali E, Erickson BR, Vincent MJ, Nichol ST, Comer JA, Rollin PE, Ksiazek TG. Crimean-Congo hemorrhagic fever in Turkey. *Emerg. Infect. Dis.* 10, 1379-84 (2004)

[37] Celikbas A, Ergonul O, Dokuzoguz B, Eren S, Baykam N, Polat-Duzgun A. Crimean Congo hemorrhagic fever infection simulating acute appendicitis. *J. Infect.* 50, 363-5 (2005)

[38] Schwarz TF, Nsanze H, Ameen AM. Clinical features of Crimean-Congo haemorrhagic fever in the United Arab Emirates. *Infection.* 25, 364-7 (1997)

[39] Suleiman MN, Muscat-Baron JM, Harries JR, Satti AG, Platt GS, Bowen ET, Simpson DI. Congo/Crimean haemorrhagic fever in Dubai. An outbreak at the Rashid Hospital. *Lancet.* 2, 939-41 (1980)

[40] Baskerville A, Satti A, Murphy FA, Simpson DI. Congo-Crimean haemorrhagic fever in Dubai: histopathological studies. *J.Clin.Pathol.* 34, 871-4 (1981)

[41] Ergonul O. Crimean-Congo haemorrhagic fever. *Lancet. Infect. Dis.* 6, 203-14 (2006)

[42] Schwarz TF, Nsanze H, Longson M, Nitschko H, Gilch S, Shurie H, Ameen A, Zahir AR, Acharya UG, Jager G. Polymerase chain reaction for diagnosis and identification of distinct variants of Crimean-Congo hemorrhagic fever virus in the United Arab Emirates. *Am. J. Trop. Med. Hyg.* 55, 190-6 (1996)

[43] Gunes T. Crimean-Congo Hemorrhagic Fever. *Mikrobiyol. Bul.* 40, 279-87 (2006)

[44] Bakir M, Ugurlu M, Dokuzoguz B, Bodur H, Tasyaran MA, Vahaboglu H; Turkish CCHF Study Group. Crimean-Congo haemorrhagic fever outbreak in Middle Anatolia: a multicentre study of clinical features and outcome measures. *J. Med. Microbiol.* 54, 385-9 (2005)

[45] Mardani M, Keshtkar-Jahromi M. Crimean-Congo hemorrhagic fever. *Arch. Iran. Med.* 10, 204-14 (2007)

[46] Flick R, Whitehouse CA.Crimean-Congo hemorrhagic fever virus. *Curr. Mol. Med.* 5, 753-60 (2005)

[47] Madani TA. Alkhumra virus infection, a new viral hemorrhagic fever in Saudi Arabia. *J. Infect.* 51, 91-7 (2005)

[48] Charrel RN, Zaki AM, Attoui H, Fakeeh M, Billoir F, Yousef AI, de Chesse R, De Micco P, Gould EA, de Lamballerie X. Complete coding sequence of the Alkhurma virus, a tick-borne flavivirus causing severe hemorrhagic fever in humans in Saudi Arabia. *Biochem. Biophys. Res. Commun.* 287, 455-61 (2001)

[49] Charrel RN, de Lamballerie X. The Alkhurma virus (family Flaviviridae, genus Flavivirus): an emerging pathogen responsible for hemorrhage fever in the Middle East. *Med. Trop. (Mars).* 63, 296-9 (2003)

[50] Charrel RN, Fagbo S, Moureau G, Alqahtani MH, Temmam S, de Lamballerie X. Alkhurma hemorrhagic fever virus in Ornithodoros savignyi ticks. *Emerg. Infect. Dis.* 13, 153-5 (2007)

[51] Charrel RN, Zaki AM, Fagbo S, de Lamballerie X. Alkhurma hemorrhagic fever virus is an emerging tick-borne flavivirus. *J. Infect.* 52, 463-4 (2006)

[52] Charrel RN, Zaki AM, Fakeeh M, Yousef AI, de Chesse R, Attoui H, de Lamballerie X. Low diversity of Alkhurma hemorrhagic fever virus, Saudi Arabia, 1994-1999. *Emerg. Infect. Dis.* 11, 683-8 (2005)

[53] Clark GG, Calisher CH, Crabbs CL, Canestorp KM, Tesh RB, Bowen RA, Taylor DE. Malpais spring virus: a new vesiculovirus from mosquitoes collected in New Mexico and evidence of infected indigenous and exotic ungulates. *Am. J. Trop. Med. Hyg.* 39, 586-92 (1988)

[54] Solomon T, Mallewa M. Dengue and other emerging flaviviruses. *J. Infect.* 42, 104-15 (2001)

[55] Volk DE, Chavez L, Beasley DW, Barrett AD, Holbrook MR, Gorenstein DG. Structure of the envelope protein domain III of Omsk hemorrhagic fever virus. *Virology.*351, 188-95 (2006)

[56] Gibbs EP, Calisher CH, Tesh RB, Lazuick JS, Bowen R, Greiner EC. Bivens arm virus: a new rhabdovirus isolated from Culicoides insignis in Florida and related to Tibrogargan virus of Australia. *Vet. Microbiol.* 19, 141-50 (1989)

[57] Tuekam T, Greiner EC, Gibbs EP. Seroepidemiology of Bivens Arm virus infections of cattle in Florida, St. Croix and Puerto Rico. *Vet. Microbiol.* 28, 121-7 (1991)

[58] Andrew M, Whiteley P, Janardhana V, Lobato Z, Gould A, Coupar B. Antigen specificity of the ovine cytotoxic T lymphocyte response to bluetongue virus. *Vet. Immunol. Immunopathol.* 47, 311-22 (1995)

[59] Inaba U. Ibaraki disease and its relationship to bluetongue. *Aust.Vet. J.* 51, 178-85 (1975)

[60] Pattnaik P. Kyasanur forest disease: an epidemiological view in India. *Rev. Med. Virol.* 16, 151-65 (2006)

[61] Pavri K. Clinical, clinicopathologic, and hematologic features of Kyasanur Forest disease. *Rev. Infect. Dis.* 11 Suppl 4, S854-9 (1989)

[62] Dandawate CN, Desai GB, Achar TR, Banerjee K. Field evaluation of formalin inactivated Kyasanur forest disease virus tissue culture vaccine in three districts of Karnataka state. *Indian. J. Med. Res.* 99, 152-8 (1994)

[63] Ghosh SN, Rajagopalan PK, Singh GK, Bhat HR. Serological evidence of arbovirus activity in birds of KFD epizootic—epidemic area, Shimoga District, Karnataka, India. *Indian. J. Med. Res.* 63, 1327-34 (1975)

[64] Goverdhan MK, Rajagopalan PK, Narasimha Murthy DP, Upadhyaya S, Boshell-M J, Trapido H, Ramachandra Rao T. Epizootiology of Kyasanur Forest Disease in wild monkeys of Shimoga district, Mysore State (1957-1964). *Indian. J. Med. Res.* 62, 497-510 (1974)

[65] Sreenivasan MA, Bhat HR, Rajagopalan PK. The epizootics of Kyasanur Forest disease in wild monkeys during 1964 to 1973. *Trans. R. Soc. Trop. Med. Hyg.* 80, 810-4 (1986)

Chapter XII

Minor Arbovirus Meningoencephalitis

Murray Valley Encephalitis

Murray Valley encephalitis is a viral encephalitis caused by the infection of the Murray Valley virus. Actually, this virus is classified within the Japanese encephalitis serocomplex of of the flavivirus type [1]. The Murray Valley encephalitis virus is an arbovirus transmitted by an arthropod, similar to many arboviruses [2]. This viral infection has emerged as an important contagious illness in the southernmost part of Asia and Australia. Trevett and Sanders said that it was important that medical doctors working in Papua New Guinea, and those who treat patients who live or work there, should aware of cases of arbovirus illness that have occurred, and the potential and the avoidable problems created by them for both the individual and the community [3].

In Australia, Murray Valley encephalitis has been reported for a long time. Historically, epidemics of a severe encephalitis occurred in eastern Australia between 1917 and 1925, in which 280 cases were reported with a mortality rate of 68%, and this unknown illness was called "Australian X" [4]. After that, the next epidemic occurred in southeast Australia in the summer of 1950–51 and the illness was given its Murray Valley encephalitis name, as this was the area in which most cases were reported [4]. This encephalitis virus was shown to be an arbovirus of the Group B (flavivirus) that was related to, but different from, Japanese encephalitis [4]. With respect to the vector of Murray Valley encephalitis, the virus is transmitted by mosquitoes, especially the *Culex* genus. The Murray Valley encephalitis virus was first detected in mosquitoes of the *annulirostris* species of *Culex* in 1960 [4]. The early seroepidemiological studies also showed that the most probable vertebrate hosts were water birds [5]. Bar et al. recently described two possible mechanisms of the introduction of this encephalitis in the epizootic regions of tropical Australia [5]. They said that isolations of the virus were done from mosquitoes, trapped shortly after the first heavy rainy season and flood in eastern Kimberley, that continued for approximately nine months into the drought [5]. They noted that Murray Valley encephalitis arose due to its introduction into viremic vertebrate hosts by mosquitoes of first generation arriving infected and continuing to take blood meals, and also to the reactivation of the virus by vertical transmission of drought-resistant eggs of *Aedes tremulus* [5]. In addition to blood-devouring *Culex annulirostris* mosquitoes, the male mosquitoes of *Aedes tremulus* are also mentioned for the action as vector for the Murray Valley encephalitis virus [5]. A hypothesis to explain the southern extension of Japanese encephalitis virus of Papua New Guinea in the islands of northern Australia in 1995 and to the Australian mainland in 1998 is the dispersion of infected mosquitoes, especially *Culex annulirostris* [6]. A similar hypothesis was proposed for Murray Valley encephalitis; nevertheless, Kay and Farrow found circumstantial evidence that air carryied toward the south approximately 200 km from Papua New Guinea to the peninsula of Cape York was possible, but that southern dispersion of Murray Valley encephalitis virus-infected mosquitoes of tropical Australia was improbable [6]. With regard to the human infection, the most recent epidemic of Murray Valley encephalitis in Australia occurred in 1974, at which time Australian encephalitis was regrouped [5]. Since 1974, nevertheless, all groups have been limited to northern Australia, especially northwestern Australia and the Kimberley region of western Australia, which contains the only confirmed foci of enzootic activity of the virus [5, 7]. In 1998, Burrow et al. carried out a study to describe the epidemiology and the clinical characteristics of Australian encephalitis in the Northern Territory of Australia between 1987 and 1996 [8]. During the period investigated, 16 patients were identified and 11 of the patients were children with distinguishing characteristics—the participation of the spinal cord and brainstem and the absence seizures in adults [8]. This can imply that young children are the majority at risk [8]. Kienzle and Small said that this encephalitis was the second serious, acute viral encephalitis to be found in Australia [9]. They noted that clinicians need to be aware of Murray Valley encephalitis in light of the growing rate of travel [9]. With regard to the neurological demonstrations in the cases with Murray Valley encephalitis, examination of CT is generally normal, and EEG does not always show focal activity [8]. Diffuse symmetrical enlargement of the thalamus and increased signs in MRI can be observed [9]. Einsiedel et al. proposed that hyperintensity T2 of the thalamus is indicative of this infection [10]. The innate resistance to flavirus infection, conferred by a single chromosome 5 locality Flv, is noted [11]. Silvia et al. carried out a study in the animal model to evaluate the resistant genetic component, Flv [11]. According to this study, Silvia et al. found that, in contrast to high viral RNA content in brains of susceptible mice, the RNA viral particle was notably reduced in the cortex, olfactory bulb, thalamus and hypothalamus of resistant mice [11]. Trace amounts of the viral RNA were detected in the medulla oblongata, while they were completely absent in the pons and cerebellum of resistant mice at different time points post infection [11]. With respect to the outcome of cases with the involvement of the CNS, the mortality and the morbidity were high [8].

Prevention of disease is attained by avoidance of mosquito exposure and vector control measures [8]. Sentinel chicken surveillance is also recommended, since human cases occurred simultaneously with chicken seroconversion in 1993 [8-9, 12].

St. Louis Encephalitis

St. Louis encephalitis is a viral encephalitis that can be found throughout North, Central, and South America and the Caribbean, and it is a major public health problem in the United

States [13-14]. Tsai noted that the periodic resurgence of epidemic outbreaks of St. Louis encephalitis was due to modifications in the environment and in human conduct contributing to changing patterns of the spreading of arboviral agents [15]. Various birds are mentioned, as important amplifying hosts in many present epidemiological reports with regard to St. Louis encephalitis [16-17]. An empirical relationship between the modeled land surface humidity and levels of human transmission of this encephalitis is also mentioned [18]. In 1980, Reefs wrote that the St. Louis encephalitis epidemics were avoidable through cautionary measures to decrease the vector [19]. Reefs described that five reciprocal factors (virus, the vector, host with viremia, human immunity and environmental temperature) were important for the epidemic [19]. Monath and Tsai noted that although a lot of progress had been made, many questions remained regarding the epidemiology and ecology of St. Louis encephalitis [19]. Various mosquitoes in the species of *Culex* are mentioned as vectors for the virus [20]. In addition to vector-borne transmission, this infection cannot be transmitted human to human, or by animal to human [20]. Shaman et al. recently analyzed the frequency of the inhibition of hemagglutination antibodies to St. Louis encephalitis in wild birds during the 1990s St. Louis encephalitis epidemic in Indian County [21]. They indicated that three factors conspired to create the 1990 epidemic: (a) a large population of susceptible wild birds; (b) the severe spring drought that facilitated the amplification of the virus between the *Culex nigripalpus* and a portion of the wild bird population; and (c) the rain continued, with resulting land surface floods in the summer and the early fall, which maintained a population of host-seeking *Culex nigripalpus* [21]. Shaman et al. concluded that the continued biting and the reproductive activity of *Culex* maintained the epizootic spread through the summer and the early fall in Indian County, and the high level of viral amplification resulted in the spread to humans [21]. Reisen et al. indicated that the persistence of protective antibodies prevented reinfection during the following season and might prevent the recrudescence of contagious virus in chronically infected birds [22].

With regard to the infection, elderly people and youth are the majority of the 30% at risk, and infected patients of advanced age will die [21]. Clinically, the symptoms of the illness begin five to 15 days after being bitten, but the majority of individuals never show any symptoms [21]. The mild cases include flu-like symptoms, with fever, headache and lethargy [21]. Severe infection generally presents with the involvement of the CNS. The neurological illness associated with acute St. Louis encephalitis includes acute aseptic meningitis, encephalomyelitis, and a poliomyelitis-like syndrome [23]. Similar to other viral encephalitis diseases, the severe cases of the virus infection can cause attacks, diplopia, paralysis and death [21]. In addition to some neurological events, few immune-mediated post-contagious events associated with the mild infection, such as encephalomyelitis, have been reported [23]. With regard to psychosocial consequences from the infection of St. Louis encephalitis, Greve et al. noted that St. Louis encephalitis produced neurocognitive deficits that were reflected in measures of psychometric as psychophysiologic and functional status [24]. They noted that psychometric and vocational improvements were observed over one year; however, the normal vocational return came at a significant psychosocial cost [24]. Although there is no evidence of congenital infection, there was a recent report on the infection in infancy [25].

Jamestown Canyon Virus Infection

Jamestown Canyon virus infection is a viral mosquito-borne disease found in America. Jamestown Canyon virus is a member of the California serogroup of family *Bunyaviridae*. Above all, it is documented in many animals, and next its importance in humans is mentioned. In 1997, Zamparo et al. determined the frequency and the virus antibody distribution in white-tailed deer (*Odocoileus virginianus*) populations in Connecticut, United States [26]. According to this study, the antibody to Jamestown Canyon virus was detected by ELISA in 21% of deer, and was evenly distributed among geographical regions [26]. Zamparo et al. concluded from this investigation and prior isolations of virus from mosquitoes in the state that Jamestown Canyon virus occured enzootically in Connecticut [26]. In 1996, Fulhorst et al. reported the first isolation of Jamestown Canyon virus in coastal California and the results of tests for the antibody to Jamestown Canyon virus in mammals that live in coastal California [27]. In this report, the isolation of the virus was made from a pool of 50 females of *Aedes dorsalis* collected as adults of Morry Bay, San Luis Obispo County, California and the isolated virus was identified by two-way plate reduction-serum dilution neutralization tests in cultures cell of VeRo [27]. According to this study, a high frequency of Jamestown Canyon virus-specific antibody was found in tested horses and cattle [27]. Fulhorst et al. said that this finding was additional evidence of the presence of an antigenically-identical or narrowly-related virus of Jamestown Canyon virus in Morry Bay, and indicated that the vectors of the virus fed from large mammals [27]. They also suggested that viruses antigenically identical or narrowly related to Jamestown Canyon virus were geographically widespread in coastal California [27].

With regard to the human infection, Jamestown Canyon virus was proposed as the etiologic agent of the widespread infection in humans in Michigan [28]. Grimstad et al. noted that in a sample population of 780 Michigan residents tested to neutralize antibodies to virus of serogroup California, 216 (27.7%) had specific neutralizing antibody to Jamestown Canyon virus [28]. They also noted that among 128 with specific neutralizing antibody to the virus, only two (1.6%) were found to have significant titers of antibody by hemagglutination inhibiting test with La Crosse virus, while 23 of 44 (52%) had significant titers with Jamestown Canyon virus; a single serum was positive for significant antibody by complement fixation tests with both viruses [28]. They proposed that complement fixation tests and tests of hemagglutination inhibition with La Crosse virus fail to detect antibody to Jamestown Canyon virus [28]. Grimstad et al. also noted that computer-drawn ASPEX maps showed that the distribution of people with antibody and residing in the southernmost part of Michigan's peninsula had a close correlation with the estimated distribution of white-tailed deer in that same part of the state, further supporting the hypothesis that those deer were the primary host of Jamestown Canyon virus [28].

With regard to the clinical demonstration of the Jamestown Canyon virus infection, the neurological manifestation is serious. A sudden onset of symptoms that begins with headache, sickness and fever that quickly progresses to the participation of central nervous system with attacks and coma is reported [29]. A concomitant rise in the complement fixation antibody to herpesvirus was also noted [29]. IgM specific antibody to Jamestown Canyon virus was useful in the diagnosis [29].

La Crosse Encephalitis

La Crosse encephalitis is an infection of arbovirus of California and is a mosquitoes-borne viral illness found in America. McJunkin et al. said that the disease is under-recognized in the United States, in spite of reports of cases in 28 states, and incidence in areas (20–30/100,000 endemic) was exceeding that of bacterial meningitis [30]. This viral mosquito-borne illness can be generally mistaken for herpes simplex encephalitis [30]. The La Crosse encephalitis virus is maintained in a cycle that implies mosquitoes and small mammals [31]. The infection of the cell of the vertebrate is generally cytolytic; the infection of the cell of vector has as a result a persistent infection [31]. This human illness is endemic in western North Carolina [32]. In 2003, Utz et al. carried out an interesting study to measure the social and economic impacts of the illness in 25 serologically confirmed encephalitis patients and/or families [32]. They found that the total direct and indirect medical costs associated with La Crosse encephalitis over 89.6 accumulated life years from the beginning of the illness to the date of interview totaled $791,374 [32]. A specific Impact of La Crosse Encephalitis Survey, or ILCES test, was utilized to measure the social impact of the infection over time for patients and families [32]. According to this study, the ILCES scores showed that the majority of the social burden of the illness was borne by the five patients with lifelong neurological sequelae [32]. Utz et al. concluded that the socioeconomic burden that resulted from the encephalitis was substantial and emphasized the importance of the illness in western North Carolina, as well as the need for the active surveillance, reporting, and programs for the prevention of the infection [2].

The La Crosse encephalitis is classified as a member the California serogroup virus (*Bunyaviridae*). Actually, many California serogroup viruses are associated with *Aedes* mosquitoes and small mammals [33]. Transovarial spreading has been demonstrated for the majority of the viruses and probably represents a greater mechanism of survival of the group [33-34]. Turell and LeDuc said that this mechanism, combined with the venereal transmission of the transovarial virus infection to uninfected females, might substantially reduce the quantity of the required amplifying vertebrate intermediates to maintain the virus in nature [33]. McJunkin et al. said that the illness occurred again each summer in endemic foci in the United States forested with hardwood trees that provided breeding grounds for the vector mosquitoes, *Aedes triseriatus* [30]. With respect to vector mosquitoes of La Crosse encephalitis, the *albopictus* species of *Aedes*, which was first identified in Houston, Texas in 1985, is an extensively-mentioned vector mosquito in the United States [35]. Public health concerns have been raised with respect to the potential of this species to serve as a vector of arboviruses to American natives, especially for La Crosse encephalitis [55].

With regard to the clinical demonstration, the clinical illness caused by La Crosse virus is generally mild. Several neurological demonstrations due to La Crosse encephalitis virus infection are mentioned. McJunkin et al. noted that La Crosse encephalitis should be considered in the boy who presented with meningoencephalitis in the summer and the early fall, and especially for children who lived in or came back from the recent trip to endemic areas in mid-Atlantic and midwestern states [31]. Rust et al. said that 30 to 180 annual cases of La Crosse encephalitis represented 8% to 30% of all cases of encephalitis in 1993 and interpretation of this common important endemic mosquitoes-borne illness in the United

States was necessary [36]. In 2001, McJunkin et al. investigated the manifestations and the clinical course of La Crosse encephalitis in 127 hospitalized patients [37]. They said that the symptoms included headache, fever, and vomiting, seizures, and confusion [37]. With regard to the demonstration of CNS, aseptic meningitis, enlargement of intracranial pressure as well as herniation of the cerebral brain could be observed [37]. In a case series, 12% of all patients had neurological deficits at discharge [37]. Follow-up evaluations showed an increase in cognitive and behavioral deficits after the episode of encephalitis [37]. Erwin et al. said that the factors significantly associated with infection of La Crosse virus included the average number of hours per day spent outdoors, living near one or more tree holes within 100 meters, and total load of *albopictus* species of *Aedes* (the number of female and male larvae and the adults collected at a site), which was around three times greater around the residences of positive La Crosse infection cases versus noncases [38]. They noted the accumulated evidence that the *Aedes albopictus* species could be implied in the outcome of La Crosse virus infection in eastern Tennessee [38]. As previously mentioned, Sokol et al. said that abnormalities of the temporal lobe of the cerebrum, commonly associated with herpes simplex encephalitis, could be observed in patients with La Crosse virus encephalitis [39]. McJunkin et al. proposed that infection of La Crosse virus should be considered in any children who presented with meningitis or aseptic encephalitis [37]. They also noted that hyponatremia and growing body temperature might be related to clinical deterioration [37]. The diagnosis was established by serologic testing for IgM and IgG antibodies of La Crosse virus [37]. The diagnostic characteristics included magnetic resonance imaging showing abnormal intensity developing in the bilateral regions of the frontotemporal lobe and periodic lateralizing epileptiform discharges [39]. Sokol et al. said that La Crosse virus encephalitis should be included in the differential diagnosis of viral encephalitis associated with structural and electrographic wounds of the temporal lobe, represented by periodic lateralizing epileptiform discharges [39]. To differentiate diagnosis of herpes simplex encephalitis, Sokol et al. said that the recently developed PCR RNA test for La Crosse virus of cerebrospinal fluid might permit rapid diagnosis, preventing the need for treatment with acyclovir, and gives parents an encouraging prognosis [39]. In comparison with another report, Hardin et al. noted that the patients with La Crosse encephalitis showed the most severe symptoms in the presentation to hospital, moreso than did patients with enteroviral-CNS infection [40]. They said that the patients with La Crosse encephalitis were significantly more likely to have aphasia, loss of consciousness, seizure, and admission to the pediatric intensive care unit. They also noted that fever, headache, vomiting, stiff neck (subjective), photophobia, behavioral changes, confusion, need for mechanical ventilation, age, and sex were not statistically significant in the course of disease [40]. Moreover, the statistical differences were not shown in the laboratory values of CSF [40]. As previously mentioned, in fact, the similarity in the profiles of CSF in different encephalitis viral disorders can be an important cause of delayed diagnosis. Neurological sequelae because of this encephalitis are comparatively rare [41]. Regarding the complications following La Crosse encephalitis, most of the neurological focal symptoms, such as the Babinski reflex, pathological reflex, aphasia, chorea, dysarthria and ataxia, resolve completely [42]. Chun said that cognitive and intellectual development of children with La Crosse encephalitis did not appear to be significantly different from that of the normal population in follow-up testing; nevertheless, there were individuals suffering from permanent damage, demonstrating lower IQ and poor academic performance [42]. Chun reported that abnormal EEG readings during the acute period were noted in 86–100% of the cases, and approximately 33% of the subjects had EEG abnormalities [42]. Nevertheless, Balkhy and Schreiber said that there was a high rate of neurological sequelae, suggesting that this infection of the CNS was not necessarily benign meningoencephalitis [41]. Chun said that recurrent seizures could occur in 6–13% of the cases one to eight years after La Crosse infection [42].

In treatment of La Crosse encephalitis, ribavirin is widely mentioned. Cassidy and Patterson said that low concentrations of ribavirin had a marked effect on the initial steps of the virus transcription [43]. A study of intravenous administration of ribavirin was led by McJunkin et al. [44]. The effectiveness of intravenous ribavirin treatment in cases of La Crosse encephalitis was noted in this study [44]. In prevention of the spread of this disease, suppression of the vector is recommended, similar to other mosquito-borne diseases. Recently, vaccination against La Crosse encephalitis was proposed as a new method for prevention of the disease. There have been many attempts to develop a DNA-based La Crosse encephalitis vaccine [45-46].

Kokobera Virus Infection

Kokobera virus is a member of the Japanese encephalitis serocomplex of this type of flavivirus [2]. This virus can be found in Australia and Papua New Guinea [47]. Poidinger et al. said that there were three topotypes of Kokobera virus: one covering Queensland and New South Wales, another represented by isolation from PNG; and a third that covered the Northern Territory and Western Australia, reported in Australia [47]. They concluded that this molecular epidemiology was significantly different from other flaviviruses in Australia, such as Murray Valley encephalitis and Kunjin virus, which are genetically unique throughout the entire Australian continent [47]. Nevertheless, Poidinger et al. said that the molecular epidemiology was similar to that of an alphavirus, Ross River virus, and this might be explained by the fact that Ross River virus utilized macropods, which had also been implied as the vertebrate host for the Kokobera virus [47]. Finally, Poidinger et al. suggested that Kokobera virus had been in the southwest of Western Australia for some time, and was not recently introduced [47]. There are some recent reports on the vector mosquitoes of Kokobera virus. The species of *Culex*, especially the *sitiens* species of *Culex* and subgroup *annulirostris*, are mentioned as an important vector of this virus [48-49]. In 2003, Johansen et al. noted that the Kokobera virus could also be isolated from *Ochlerotatus vigilax* [48]. Van Den Hurk et al. mentioned the importance of the co-presence of other flaviviruses in the vector mosquitoes [49]. The clinical manifestation of Kokobera virus infection, nevertheless, at the time of infection is usually presumptively identified as dengue fever infection [50].

Eastern Equine Encephalitis

Eastern equine encephalitis is a mosquitoes-borne infection disease. The causative agent is this illness is a member of *Togaviridae*. This illness is above all described in the horse; nevertheless, it emerges as a human infection later. The vector mosquitoes are *Culiseta melanura, Coquillettidia pertubans*, and *Aedes vexans*. The birds are considered an important component in the spreading of this illness. In 2003, Cupp et al. carried out an interesting study to investigate the transmission of this equine encephalomyelitis virus in central Alabama [51]. In this study, five species of mosquitoes—*Culiseta melanura, Coquillettidia pertubans, Aedes vexans, Culex erraticus* and *Uranotaenia sapphirina*—were examined for the presence of virus utilizing an RT-PCR test for the eastern equine encephalitis virus [51]. Cupp et al. found that *Culiseta melanura* was a probable endemic vector in central Alabama, while *Coquillettidia pertubans* and *Aedes vexans* probably functioned as bridging vectors [51]. In 2004, Garvin et al. carried out a serosurvey on avians for the virus in Killbuck Marsh Wildlife (KMWA), a focus of the infection in central Ohio [52]. They suggested that dry conditions reduced the breeding and abundance of *Culiseta melanura* and possibly the spread of eastern equine encephalitis in KMWA [52]. Of interest, Cupp et al. said that *Uranotaenia sapphirina* was considered to be feeding off amphibians and possibly reptilians, which were also found to carry the virus, and suggested that other species such as birds might serve as a reservoir for this encephalitis virus in hardwood swamps in the United States, especially in the southeast and nearby areas [51]. Cupp et al. said that species of ectothermic hosts were possible eastern equine encephalitis virus reservoirs in the southeastern United States, where species such as *Culex peccator* and *Uranotaenia sapphirina* occurred in large diverse reptilian, amphibian and avian populations [53].

Eastern equine encephalitis mainly occurs on the east and gulf coasts of the United States [54]. Deresiewicz et al. reviewed all human cases of reported eastern equine encephalitis in the United States between 1988 and 1994 and found that the mortality rate was 36%, and 35% of the survivors were moderately or severely incapacitated [54]. With regard to the clinical demonstrations, a patient with this encephalitis generally presents with fever and altered mental status, and has focal cranial lesions that are evident in both computed tomography (CT) and MRI [54-55]. Nevertheless, the alterations in the CNS can be observed [55]. Deresiewicz et al. noted that those abnormalities of neuroradiographic findings were common, and radiographic demonstrations of this viral encephalitis could be better represented, in the early phase, by MRI [54]. With regard to neuroimaging, common abnormal conclusions are generally focal lesions in basal ganglia, thalami, and in the brain stem, while cortical lesions, meningeal enhancement, and changes of the periventricular white-matter are less common [54]. Deresiewicz et al. said that the characteristic early involvement of the basal ganglia and thalami in this illness distinguish it from herpes simplex encephalitis [54]. Deresiewicz et al. proposed that the presence of large radiographical lesions did not predict a poor outcome, but high cerebrospinal fluid white cell counts or severe hyponatremia did [54].

Western Equine Encephalitis

Western equine encephalitis is a mosquito-borne infectious disease. The causative agent is either Venezuelan equine encephalitis virus or western equine enchephalitis virus, which are members of *Togaviridae*. Similar to eastern equine encephalitis, this disease was first described in the horse; however, it later became an emerging human infection. This disease is also a significant problem for many farm animals and fowl. The illness can be seen in the United States and in Latin America. The mosquito vectors are species of *Culex* mosquitoes, especially *tarsalis* species. In the human, Roman-Lieber and Iversson carried out an investigation of serological parameters in arbovirus infections in residents of an ecological reserve in Brazil and they found an intense circulation of pathogenic arboviruses, especially Venezuelan equine encephalitis virus [56]. They noted also that the habit of entering the forest was the most important factor to the exposure of the population to the vectors of many arboviruses including Venezualan equine encephalitis and western equine enchephalitis [56]. Similar to eastern equine enchephalitis, birds are mentioned for their important role in the transmisison of western equine encephalitis. According to an investigation of the seroprevalence among birds in California, Reisen et al. found that House finches, house sparrows, Gambel's quail, California quail, common ground doves, and mourning doves were most frequently positive for antibodies [57]. Reisen et al. noted that the initial discovery of enzootic activity each summer closely coincided with the appearance to hatching birds in the areas of the study, indicating their role in the amplification of the virus [57]. They also proposed that normally positive species of bird roosted or nested in the elevated upland vegetation, places where host-seeking *Culex tarsalis* females normally hunt [57]. Various outbreaks of Venezualan equine encephalitis were reported in humans and horses in South America and the United States, especially in the southern part [58-59]. This virus generally causes a feverish illness that might be complicated with encephalitis, mainly in the cases of children and patients of advanced age [58]. For diagnosis of the infection in humans, several serological tests, including neutralizing, hemagglutination inhibiting and complement-fixation, are available [60]. With regard to the pathology of CNS due to the infection of this virus, focal neurological signs are reported [61]. The pathological conclusions include perivascular infiltrates and multifocal necrosis in the deep gray matter, ganglia and basal spinal cord [61].

Tick Borne Encephalitis

Tick borne encephalitis (TBE), or Powassan encephalitisis, is an arboviral (flaviviral type) encephalitis in which the tick is the main vector. It is a viral zoonosis transmitted by infected ticks harboring the TBE virus [62]. The mortality rate can reach 30%. More than 10,000 patients were reported annually in Europe and Far East Asia [62]. This disease has been known for many decades. In Finland, TBE has been observed in the Aland Islands (population 26,500) for more than 60 years [63]. The annual number of patients has ranged from 1 to 26, and has increased over time. The clinical picture has not undergone any conspicuous changes [63]. It is believed that TBE is the most important flaviviral infection of the CNS in Europe and Russia [64]. The Siberian subtype of TBE, which is predominant in Russia, circulated continuously in eastern European regions for six decades and in the Urals and west and east Siberia for six decades [65]. Similar to the situation in Finland, changes were not found in the structure of viral populations at the peak and drop of the incidence of TBE [65].

Concerning the vectors of TBE, *Ixodes* species are the main tick vectors. These ticks are characterized by a comparatively long life cycle, lasting several years, during which the infecting virus may be maintained from one developmental stage of the tick to the next [65-67]. *Ixodes ricinis* is the main vector for most TBE cases. For the Siberian subtype, two types of ticks, *Ixodes persulcatus* and *Ixodes ricinis*, are the main vectors. The *Ixodes ricinus* tick has been recorded in most European regions, especially in thermo-mesophilous woods and shrubby habitats where the relative humidity allow the tick to complete its three-year developmental cycle, as predicted for the European climatic ranges [66]. Rodents and roe deer (*Capreolus capreolus*) are the wildlife reservoirs that play a central role in the persistence of these infections [66]. The dynamics of transmission are as follows: a) in the tick, following virus uptake in the infected blood meal, infection of the midgut, passage through the hemocoel to the salivary glands, and transmission via the saliva; and b) in the vertebrate host, virus delivery into the skin at the site of tick feeding, infection of the draining lymph nodes, and dissemination to target organs [67]. It is found that proteins and other chemicals, secreted in tick saliva, control the vertebrate hosts' haemostatic, inflammatory and immune responses in order to facilitate blood-feeding [68]. Such bioactive saliva molecules include immunoglobulin-binding proteins, histamine-binding proteins, natural killer cells and interferon regulators, and complement inhibitors [68]. In addition, it can also be transmitted by the ingestion of raw goat milk.

Classically, boundaries of the virus range and the location of natural foci within it are closely associated with the distribution pattern of these ticks [69]. However, a currently observed marked increased incidence of various tick borne diseases in many parts of Europe is due to documented climatic changes as well anthropogenic influence on habitat structure [70]. Zajkowska et al. said that spring temperatures above 7–10 degrees C allow the nymphs and larvae of *Ixodes ricinus* to feed simultaneously on rodents [70].

Concerning clinical presentation, TBE is a benign self-limiting illness that usually resolves without any reliquiae [71]. According to the data from Finland [63], a few patients have had permanent neurological damage. This can confirm the benign nature of TBE. However, this data seems to be different from other European countries. The lethality of TBE in Europe is 0.5%, and a post-encephalitic syndrome is seen in more than 40% of affected patients, often producing a pronounced impairment in quality of life [64]. The laboratory diagnosis is obtained by isolating the virus in cell cultures from the CSF or blood of acute-phase patients. Serology is the main laboratory tool to perform this diagnosis [71]. Complement fixation and EIA IgM are the most used methods: the latter technique is particularly sensitive in early infection [71]. Neurological signs and symptoms can be seen in a few cases. If the nervous system is affected, four clinical features of different severity can be observed: meningitis, meningoencephalitis, meningoencephalomyelitis, meningoradiculoneuritis [72]. A direct comparison of the course and outcome of TBE revealed several distinctions between patients over 60 years of age and those aged 60 or under and corroborates previous assumptions that TBE is a more serious illness in the elderly population [73]. Treatment for cases of TBE with neurological symptoms consists of symptomatic treatment similar to other arboviral meningoencephalitis. No effective drug is available at present.

TBE is a preventable disease, which is rapidly becoming a growing public health problem in Europe [72]. So far no causal treatment is possible, but an efficient, safe vaccination is available [72]. Until the present, active immunization is the only reliable means of preventing TBE [74]. Evidence suggests that effectiveness is greater than 95% [74].

Vaccines to protect against TBE are produced by two manufacturers and are widely used in European and Asian countries, where TBE virus is endemic [75]. General trends in vaccine development during recent decades and extensive postmarketing experience resulted in several modifications to their formulations and practical implications for use [75]. Prolonged immunity after the vaccination can be observed; therefore, the current practice of administering booster doses every three years is a topic of intense debate [74]. A prolongation of booster intervals at least in younger adults is proposed by Rendi-Wagner et al. [76]. Recommendations for prolongation of TBE booster intervals have been made in several European countries, and a concensus for booster recommendations is predicted within the European Union [75]. A common question that is frequently asked regarding these two vaccines concerns their exchangeability [77]. Broker and Schondorf suggested boosting or continuation of uncompleted primary immunization schedules with either of the two tick-borne encephalitis vaccines [77]. Recently, new vaccines have become available, the most modern versions of which do not contain the commonly used protein-derived stabilizers (human albumin or polygeline) of former vaccines [78]. Post-marketing experience supports results from clinical trials showing that these new TBE vaccines may safely be used for the vaccination of children, adolescents, and adults [78]. Of interest, Austria is the country with the highest coverage of TBE vaccination (86% of the total population) and this has led to a dramatic reduction in the annual number of clinical cases and proves under field conditions that vaccination is an effective means for the prophylaxis of TBE [79-80].

References

[1] Poidinger M, Hall RA, Mackenzie JS. Molecular characterization of the Japanese encephalitis serocomplex of the flavivirus genus. *Virology*. 218, 417-21 (1996)

[2] Solomon T, Mallewa M. Dengue and other emerging flaviviruses. *J. Infect.* 42, 104-15 (2001)

[3] Trevett AJ, Sanders RC. Arbovirus disease in Papua New Guinea. *P. N. G. Med J.* 37, 116-24 (1994)

[4] Mackenzie JS, Broom AK. Australian X disease, Murray Valley encephalitis and the French connection. *Vet. Microbiol.* 46, 79-90 (1995)

[5] Broom AK, Lindsay MD, Johansen CA, Wright AE, Mackenzie JS. Two possible mechanisms for survival and initiation of Murray Valley encephalitis virus activity in the Kimberley region of Western Australia. *Am. J. Trop. Med. Hyg.* 53, 95-9 (1995)

[6] Kay BH, Farrow RA. Mosquitoes (Diptera: Culicidae) dispersal: implications for the epidemiology of Japanese and Murray Valley encephalitis viruses in Australia. *J. Med. Entomol.* 37, 797-801 (2000)

[7] Russell RC. Mosquitoes-borne arboviruses in Australia: the current scene and implications of climate change for human health. *Int. J. Parasitol.* 28, 955-69(1998)

[8] Burrow JN, Whelan PI, Kilburn CJ, Fisher DA, Currie BJ, Smith DW. Australian encephalitis in the Northern Territory: clinical and epidemiological features, 1987-1996. *Aust. N. Z. J. Med.* 28, 590-6 (1998)

[9] Kienzle N, Boyes L. Murray Valley encephalitis: case report and review of neuroradiological features. *Australas. Radiol.* 47, 61-3 (2003)

[10] Einsiedel L, Kat E, Ravindran J, Slavotinek J, Gordon DL. MR findings in Murray Valley encephalitis. AJNR *Am. J. Neuroradiol.* 24, 1379-82 (2003)

[11] Silvia OJ, Pantelic L, Mackenzie JS, Shellam GR, Papadimitriou J, Urosevic N. Virus spread, tissue inflammation and antiviral response in brains of flavivirus susceptible and resistant mice acutely infected with Murray Valley encephalitis virus. *Arch. Virol.* 149, 447-64 (2004)

[12] Broom AK. Sentinel Chicken Surveillance Program in Australia, July 2002 to June 2003. *Commun. Dis. Intell.* 27, 367-9(2003)

[13] Vector borne diseases. Available at http://www.fpnotebook.com/ID211.htm

[14] Changes in the Incidence of Vector-Borne Diseases Attributable to Climate Change. Available at http://www.ciesin.org/TG/HH/veclev2.html

[15] Tsai TF. Arboviral infections in the United States. *Infect. Dis. Clin. North. Am.* 5, 73-102 (1991)

[16] Reisen WK. Epidemiology of St. Louis encephalitis virus. *Adv. Virus. Res.* 61, 139-83 (2003)

[17] Lord CC, Day JF. Simulation studies of St. Louis encephalitis and West Nile viruses: the impact of bird mortality. *Vector. Borne. Zoonotic. Dis.* 1, 317-29 (2001)

[18] Shaman J, Day JF, Stieglitz M. St. Louis encephalitis virus in wild birds during the 1990 south Florida epidemic: the importance of drought, wetting conditions, and the emergence of Culex nigripalpus (Diptera: Culicidae) to arboviral amplification and transmission. *J. Med. Entomol.* 40, 547-54 (2003)

[19] Shaman J, Day JF, Stieglitz M, Zebiak S, Cane M. Seasonal forecast of St. Louis encephalitis virus transmission, Florida. *Emerg, Infect, Dis.* 10, 802-9 (2004)

[20] Monath TP, Tsai TF. St. Louis encephalitis: lessons from the last decade. *Am. J. Trop. Med. Hyg.* 37(3 Suppl), 40S-59S (1987)

[21] Ruby JP. St. Louis encephalitis. *Epidemiol. Rev.* 1, 55-73 (1979)

[22] Reisen WK, Chiles RE, Green EN, Fang Y, Mahmood F. Previous infection protects house finches from re-infection with St. Louis encephalitis virus. *J. Med. Entomol.* 40, 300-5 (2003)

[23] Sejvar JJ, Bode AV, Curiel M, Marfin AA. Post-infectious encephalomyelitis associated with St. Louis encephalitis virus infection. *Neurology.* 63, 1719-21 (2004)

[24] Greve KW, Houston RJ, Adams D, Stanford MS, Bianchini KJ, Clancy A, Rabito FJ Jr. The neurobehavioural consequences of St. Louis encephalitis infection. *Brain. Inj.* 16, 917-27 (2002)

[25] Wootton SH, Kaplan SL, Perrotta DM, Martin DA, Campbell GL. St. Louis encephalitis in early infancy. *Pediatr. Infect. Dis J.* 23, 951-4 (2004)

[26] Zamparo JM, Andreadis TG, Shope RE, Tirrell SJ. Serologic evidence of Jamestown Canyon virus infection in white-tailed deer populations from Connecticut. *J. Wildl. Dis.* 33, 623-7 (1997)

[27] Fulhorst CF, Hardy JL, Eldridge BF, Chiles RE, Reeves WC. Ecology of Jamestown Canyon virus (Bunyaviridae: California serogroup) in coastal California. *Am. J. Trop. Med. Hyg.* 55, 185-9 (1996)

[28] Grimstad PR, Calisher CH, Harroff RN, Wentworth BB. Jamestown Canyon virus (California serogroup) is the etiologic agent of widespread infection in Michigan humans. *Am. J. Trop. Med. Hyg.* 35, 376-86 (1986)

[29] Grimstad PR, Shabino CL, Calisher CH, Waldman RJ. A case of encephalitis in a human associated with a serologic rise to Jamestown Canyon virus. *Am. J. Trop. Med. Hyg.* 31, 1238-44 (1982)

[30] McJunkin JE, Khan RR, Tsai TF. California-La Crosse encephalitis. *Infect. Dis. Clin. North. Am.* 12, 83-93 (1998)

[31] Borucki MK, Kempf BJ, Blitvich BJ, Blair CD, Beaty BJ. La Crosse virus: replication in vertebrate and invertebrate hosts. *Microbes. Infect.* 4, 341-50 (2002)

[32] Utz JT, Apperson CS, MacCormack JN, Salyers M, Dietz EJ, McPherson JT. Economic and social impacts of La Crosse encephalitis in western North Carolina. *Am. J. Trop. Med. Hyg.* 69, 509-18 (2003)

[33] Turell MJ, LeDuc JW. The role of mosquitoes in the natural history of California serogroup viruses. *Prog. Clin. Biol. Res.* 123, 43-55 (1983)

[34] Eldridge BF. Evolutionary relationships among California serogroup viruses (Bunyaviridae) and Aedes mosquitoeses (Diptera: Culicidae). *J. Med. Entomol.* 27, 738-49(1990)

[35] Francy DB, Moore CG, Eliason DA. Past, present and future of Aedes albopictus in the United States. *J. Am. Mosq. Control. Assoc.* 6, 127-32 (1990)

[36] Rust RS, Thompson WH, Matthews CG, Beaty BJ, Chun RW. La Crosse and other forms of California encephalitis. *J. Child. Neurol.* 14, 1-14 (1999)

[37] McJunkin JE, de los Reyes EC, Irazuzta JE, Caceres MJ, Khan RR, Minnich LL, Fu KD, Lovett GD, Tsai T, Thompson A. La Crosse encephalitis in children. *N. Engl. J. Med.* 344, 801-7 (2001)

[38] Erwin PC, Jones TF, Gerhardt RR, Halford SK, Smith AB, Patterson LE, Gottfried KL, Burkhalter KL, Nasci RS, Schaffner W. La Crosse encephalitis in Eastern Tennessee: clinical, environmental, and entomological characteristics from a blinded cohort study. *Am. J. Epidemiol.* 155, 1060-5 (2002)

[39] Sokol DK, Kleiman MB, Garg BP. LaCrosse viral encephalitis mimics herpes simplex viral encephalitis. *Pediatr. Neurol.* 25, 413-5 (2001)

[40] Hardin SG, Erwin PC, Patterson L, New D, Graber C, Halford SK. Clinical comparisons of La Crosse encephalitis and enteroviral central nervous system infections in a pediatric population: 2001 surveillance in East Tennessee. *Am. J. Infect. Control.* 3, 508-10 (2003)

[41] Balkhy HH, Schreiber JR. Severe La Crosse encephalitis with significant neurologic sequelae. *Pediatr. Infect. Dis. J.* 19, 77-80 (2000)

[42] Chun RW. Clinical aspects of La Crosse encephalitis: neurological and psychological sequelae. *Prog. Clin. Biol. Res.* 123, 193-201 (1983)

[43] Cassidy LF, Patterson JL. Mechanism of La Crosse virus inhibition by ribavirin. *Antimicrob. Agents. Chemother.* 33, 2009-11 (1989)

[44] McJunkin JE, Khan R, de los Reyes EC, Parsons DL, Minnich LL, Ashley RG, Tsai TF. Treatment of severe La Crosse encephalitis with intravenous ribavirin following diagnosis by brain biopsy. *Pediatrics.* 99, 261-7 (1997)

[45] Pavlovic J, Schultz J, Hefti HP, Schuh T, Molling K. DNA vaccination against La Crosse virus. *Intervirology.* 43, 312-21 (2000)

[46] Schuh T, Schultz J, Moelling K, Pavlovic J. DNA-based vaccine against La Crosse virus: protective immune response mediated by neutralizing antibodies and CD4+ T cells. *Hum. Gene. Ther.* 10,1649-58 (1999)

[47] Poidinger M, Hall RA, Lindsay MD, Broom AK, Mackenzie JS. The molecular epidemiology of Kokobera virus. *Virus. Res.* 68, 7-13 (2000)

[48] Johansen CA, Nisbet DJ, Zborowski P, van den Hurk AF, Ritchie SA, Mackenzie JS. Flavivirus isolations from mosquitoeses collected from western Cape York Peninsula, Australia, 1999-2000. *J. Am. Mosq. Control. Assoc.* 19, 392-6 (2003)

[49] Van Den Hurk AF, Johansen CA, Zborowski P, Phillips DA, Pyke AT, Mackenzie JS, Ritchie SA. Flaviviruses isolated from mosquitoeses collected during the first recorded outbreak of Japanese encephalitis virus on Cape York Peninsula, Australia. *Am. J. Trop. Med. Hyg.* 64, 125-30. (2001)

[50] Mein J, O'Grady KA, Whelan P, Merianos A. Dengue or Kokobera? A case report from the top end of the Northern Territory. *Commun. Dis. Intell.* 105-7.(1998)

[51] Cupp EW, Klingler K, Hassan HK, Viguers LM, Unnasch TR. Transmission of eastern equine encephalomyelitis virus in central Alabama. *Am. J. Trop. Med. Hyg.* 68, 495-500 (2003)

[52] Garvin MC, Ohajuruka OA, Bell KE, Ives SL. Seroprevalence of eastern equine encephalomyelitis virus in birds and larval survey of Culiseta melanura Coquillett during an interepizootic period in central Ohio. *J. Vector. Ecol.* 29, 73-8 (2004)

[53] Cupp EW, Zhang D, Yue X, Cupp MS, Guyer C, Sprenger TR, Unnasch TR. Identification of reptilian and amphibian blood meals from mosquitoeses in an eastern equine encephalomyelitis virus focus in central Alabama. *Am. J. Trop. Med. Hyg.* 71, 272-6 (2004)

[54] Deresiewicz RL, Thaler SJ, Hsu L, Zamani AA. Clinical and neuroradiographic manifestations of eastern equine encephalitis. *N. Engl. J. Med.* 336, 1867-74 (1997)

[55] Piliero PJ, Brody J, Zamani A, Deresiewicz RL. Eastern equine encephalitis presenting as focal neuroradiographic abnormalities: case report and review. *Clin. Infect. Dis.* 18, 985-8 (1994)

[56] Romano-Lieber NS, Iversson LB. Serological survey on arbovirus infection in residents of an ecological reserve. *Rev. Saude. Publica.* 34, 236-42 (2000)

[57] Reisen WK, Lundstrom JO, Scott TW, Eldridge BF, Chiles RE, Cusack R, Martinez VM, Lothrop HD, Gutierrez D, Wright SE, Boyce K, Hill BR. Patterns of avian

seroprevalence to western equine encephalomyelitis and Saint Louis encephalitis viruses in California, USA. *J. Med. Entomol.* 37, 507-27 (2000)

[58] Stienlauf S, Eisenkraft A, Robenshtok E, Hourvitz A. Viral encephalitis caused by biowarfare agents. *Harefuah.* 141 Spec No, 51-6 (2002)

[59] Calisher CH. Medically important arboviruses of the United States and Canada. *Clin. Microbiol. Rev.* 7, 89-116 (1994)

[60] Boctor FN, Calisher CH, Peter JB. Dot-ELISA for serodiagnosis of human infections due to Western equine encephalitis virus. *J. Virol. Methods.* 26, 305-11 (1989)

[61] Anderson BA. Focal neurologic signs in western equine encephalitis. *Can. Med. Assoc. J.* 130, 1019-21 (1984)

[62] Takashima I. Tick-borne encephalitis. *Nippon. Rinsho.* 63, 2202-6 (2005)

[63] Wahlberg P, Carlsson SA, Granlund H, Jansson C, Linden M, Nyberg C, Nyman D. TBE in Aland Islands 1959-2005: Kumlinge disease. *Scand. J. Infect. Dis.* 38, 1057-62 (2006)

[64] Gunther G, Haglund M. Tick-borne encephalopathies : epidemiology, diagnosis, treatment and prevention. *CNS. Drugs.* 19, 1009-32 (2005)

[65] Pogodina VV. Monitoring of tick-borne encephalitis virus populations and etiological structure of morbidity over 60 years. *Vopr. Virusol.* 50, 7-13 (2005)

[66] Rizzoli A, Rosa R, Mantelli B, Pecchioli E, Hauffe H, Tagliapietra V, Beninati T, Neteler M, Genchi C. Ixodes ricinus, transmitted diseases and reservoirs. *Parassitologia.* 46, 119-22 (2004)

[67] Nuttall PA, Labuda M. Dynamics of infection in tick vectors and at the tick-host interface. *Adv. Virus. Res.* 60, 233-72 (2003)

[68] Nuttall PA. Pathogen-tick-host interactions: Borrelia burgdorferi and TBE virus. *Zentralbl. Bakteriol.* 289, 492-505 (1999)

[69] Korenberg EI, Kovalevskii YV. Main features of tick-borne encephalitis eco-epidemiology in Russia. *Zentralbl. Bakteriol.* 289, 525-39 (1999)

[70] Zajkowska J, Malzahn E, Kondrusik M, Grygorczuk S, Pancewicz SS, Kusmierczyk J, Czupryna P, Hermanowska-Szpakowicz T. Tick borne encephalitis and enviromental changes. Przegl Epidemiol. 60 Suppl 1, 186-9, 191 (2006)

[71] Sambri V, Marangoni A, Storni E, Cavrini F, Moroni A, Sparacino M, Cevenini R. Tick borne zoonosis: selected clinical and diagnostic aspects. *Parassitologia.* 46, 109-13 (2004)

[72] Kunze U, Asokliene L, Bektimirov T, Busse A, Chmelik V, Heinz FX, Hingst V, Kadar F, Kaiser R, Kimmig P, Kraigher A, Krech T, Linquist L, Lucenko I, Rosenfeldt V, Ruscio M, Sandell B, Salzer H, Strle F, Suss J, Zilmer K, Mutz I. Tick-borne encephalitis in childhood--consensus 2004. *Wien. Med. Wochenschr.* 154, 242-5 (2004)

[73] Logar M, Bogovic P, Cerar D, Avsic-Zupanc T, Strle F. Tick-borne encephalitis in Slovenia from 2000 to 2004: comparison of the course in adult and elderly patients. *Wien. Klin. Wochenschr.* 118, 702-7 (2006)

[74] Aebi C. Prevention of tick-borne encephalitis (TBE). *Ther. Umsch.* 62, 726-30 (2005)

[75] Zent O, Broker M. Tick-borne encephalitis vaccines: past and present. *Expert. Rev. Vaccines.* 4, 747-55 (2005)

[76] Rendi-Wagner P, Zent O, Jilg W, Plentz A, Beran J, Kollaritsch H. Persistence of antibodies after vaccination against tick-borne encephalitis. *Int. J. Med. Microbiol.* 296 Suppl 40, 202-7 (2006)

[77] Broker M, Schondorf I. Are tick-borne encephalitis vaccines interchangeable? *Expert. Rev. Vaccines.* 5, 461-6 (2006)

[78] Zent O, Hennig R, Banzhoff A, Broker M. Tick-borne encephalitis vaccines: past and present. Expert. Rev. Vaccines. 4, 747-55 (2005)

[79] Heinz FX, Kunz C. Tick-borne encephalitis and the impact of vaccination. *Arch. Virol. Suppl.* 18, 201-5 (2004)

[80] Kunz C. Vaccination against TBE in Austria: the success story continues. *Int. J. Med. Microbiol.* 291 Suppl 33, 56-7 (2002)

Chapter XIII

Minor Arbovirus Arthritis

Ross River Virus Infection

Ross River virus is a mosquito-borne viral infection. This arthritides is important in a public health sense and is responsible for a far greater number of infections [1]. The Ross River virus is a mosquito-borne arbovirus that is widely responsible for many outbreaks of polyarthritis illness throughout Australia. Russell et al. noted that the case reports of Ross River virus infection totaled approximately 30,000 during 1991–1996 [1]. In 2005, Harley et al. utilized a prospective matched case-control study of new cases of this infection in local government areas of Marimba, of Douglas, and of Atherton in tropical Queensland [2]. Harley et al. said that protective measures against mosquitoes reduced the risk of illnesses, and mosquito repellents and citronela candles each diminished the risk at least two fold, with a dose-response for the number of utilized protective measures [2]. Kelly-Hope et al. analyzed a century of historical data of outbreaks of Ross River viral illness and found that although high Southern Oscillation Index and La Nina conditions were potentially important predictors of outcome in the Murray Darling River region, this was not true for the other four ecological zones in Australia where Ross River virus infections were reported [3]. They noted other factors that contribute to the emergence of the Ross River virus infection in Australia [3]. Kelly-Hope et al. compared monthly and seasonal tendencies of rain and temperature in years of outbreak in four non-outbreak epidemic-prone locations [4]. They found that climatic differences occurred between years of outbreak and non-outbreak; nevertheless, seasonal and monthly trends differed among geo-climatic regions of the country [4].

With regard to clinical manifestations, this infection is an illness whose symptoms are arthritis, arthralgia, lethargy, rash and fever that can persist for weeks or months. Recently, Condon and Rouse carried out a retrospective study to describe the nature and duration of symptoms of the Ross River virus infection in Western Australia, and in the related functional disability, to determine the perceived efficacy of treatment and to determine the usefulness of available information on the Ross River virus infection [5]. In this series, the most common symptoms were arthralgia, exhaustion and lethargy, and joint inflexibility and swelling [5]. In patients with joint manifestations, knees, wrists and ankles were almost always affected [5]. Condon and Rouse said that non-steroidal anti-inflammatory agents, rest, analgesics and simple hydrotherapy were subjectively the most useful treatments [5]. Condon and Rouse noted that people infected with Ross River virus in the southwestern part of Western Australia, compared with patients in another part of Australia, experienced a slightly different spectrum of clinical symptoms with a longer period of incapacity, and this might be related to the presence of a topotype difference from the virus found in another part of Australia [5]. Condon and Rouse said that there was no indication that arthritides of alphaviral infection predisposed to other conditions; thus, the patients whose Ross River virus illness was actually resolved might be diagnosed with other conditions [6]. They also noted that polyarthritis of Ross River virus probably arose from the associated inflammation with productive viral infections in synovial macrophages that persisted in spite of neutralizing antibodies and the antiviral responses of cytokines, and the persistence might be facilitated by downregulation of responses of cytokines by the virus-antibody complexes that are tied to receivers of Fc and induction of interleukin-10 [6]. The early discovery of the increased activity of the virus in populations of mosquitoes permits public health authorities to apply measures to reduce the number of human infections during epidemics [7]. The present surveillance techniques require a minimum of four weeks for the virus to be isolated and to be identified [7]. Therefore, there are several new investigative attempts to develop instruments for the discovery of the infection. Oliveira et al. reported that the use of enzyme immunoassays (EIA) provided a specific, sensitive, and fast alternative to traditional methods for the virus detection in vector mosquitoes [7]. With respect to the diagnosis of the infection in humans, this infection can be diagnosed by a specific serological test. Recently, Sellner et al. tested PCR for diagnosis and found that while PCR could not replace serology for Ross River virus diagnosis, it might be useful in conjunction with serological testing, especially to form a final diagnos in those samples with low titers not decisive of antibody [8]. They proposed that these tests were faster and more sensitive than isolation of virus by laboratory culture, and they would be able to show usefulness in investigations of the pathogenesis of the illness [8].

Barmah Forest Virus Infection

Barmah Forest virus infection is a mosquito-borne arboviral infection. This arthritides has become an important public health matter in Australia [1]. There have been various extensively separated outbreaks in the Barmah Forest in recent years, and reports of cases increase yearly [1]. The activity of the virus is widespread but often is localized, driven mainly by an abundance of mosquitoes, and several species are implied; host factors are also implied, but they are not well understood [1]. In 2000, Boyd and Key studied the competence of vectors of *aegypti* species of *Aedes*, *sitiens* species of *Culex*, *annulirostris* species of *Culex*, and *quinquefasciatus* species of *Culex* for the Barmah Forest virus [9]. They found that only *annulirostris* species of *Culex* was susceptible to the infection, and transmission of the virus to suckling mice by *Culex annulirostris* occurred two days after infection [9]. They also noted that transmission of *Culex annulirostris* was 10% two days after infection and did not exceed 8% thereafter [9]. Boyd and Key concluded that although *Culex annulirostris* could be infected and were capable of transmitting Barmah Forest virus to mice, it was nevertheless a relatively ineffective vector of the virus [9]. Doggett et al. said that the largest registered outbreak of human illness resulting from mosquito transmission of the alphavirus Barmah Forest virus occurred along the southern coast of New South Wales, Australia in 1995 [10]. Historically, the virus was first isolated at the beginning of January from mosquitoes collected at Batemans Bay [10]. *Aedes vigilax* was the suspected vector mosquito in this outbreak [10]. Doggett et al. noted that the outbreak of Barmah Forest virus appeared to be associated with various factors, and they proposed that a lack of recent activity of Barmah Forest virus in the region provided an extremely susceptible human population, and the exceptional conditions of above-average rain matched with high tides resulted in an increase in populations of *vigilax* species of *Aedes* [10].

With regard to a similar viral encephalitis infection, the clinical manifestations of Ross River virus infection are arthritis and arthralgia. Barmah Forest viral exanthem, presenting with eruptions characterized by erythema of urticated lesions with the most minimum epidermal change, is also reported [11]. Flexman et al. said that arthritis was more common and more prominent in the Ross River virus infection, and rash was more common and florid with the Barmah Forest virus infection, although the illnesses could not be definitively distinguished by the clinical symptoms [12]. With respect to diagnosis of the infection in the human, this infection can be definitely diagnosed by a specific serological test [11-12]. Flexman et al. said that arthralgia, myalgia and lethargy might continue for at least six months in half of patients with Ross River virus infection, but in only about 10% of patients with the Barmah Forest virus infection [12]. Similar to the infection of Ross River virus, management of symptoms is recommended for infection of Barmah Forest virus [12].

Sindbis Virus Infection, or Pogosta Disease

Sindbis virus is an arthritis-causing arbovirus [13]. Sindbis virus is widespread in Europe, Africa, Australia, and Asia, but clinical infection occurs as epidemic in a few geographically restricted areas [14]. Sindbis virus causes Pogosta disease, a mosquito-borne viral disease, which is clinically manifested by rash and arthritis. Kurkela et al. reported that the typical symptoms during the acute phase of Pogosta disease were arthritis, itching rash, fatigue, mild fever, headache, and muscle pain [14]. The most notable finding was that, in 50% of the patients, joint symptoms lasted for >12 months [14]. Detection of the virus in blood and skin lesions can help diagnosis [15]. Laine et al. reported that Sindbis virus infection might be associated with either acute joint inflammation as a part of Pogosta disease or chronic arthritis [16]. Turunen et al. reported clinical observations during an outbreak of Pogosta disease in the province of North Karelia, Finland [17]. According to this case series, the main manifestations were fever (23%), rash (88%) and joint symptoms (93%) [17]. The joint symptoms in some patients lasted for several months and were severe enough to cause immobilization [17]. Brummer-Korvenkontio et al. found that the depth of snow cover and the temperature in May–July seemed to predict the number of cases [18]. They also reported that the morbidity was highest in 45- to 65-year-old females and lowest in children [18]. Of interest, Sindbis virus and other alphavirus gene expression vectors have recently been used to express and study the functions of proteins and RNA, to evaluate classical vaccine and novel antiviral approaches, and for nucleic acid immunization [19]. A recent report demonstrates that the Sindbis virus has remarkable properties in three challenging areas of gene therapy including specificity, efficacy and delivery, suggesting that Sindbis has the potential to become an important gene therapy vector for cancer therapy [20].

Sindbis-related Ockelbo or Karelian fever viruses have been found to cause significant morbidity [13]. The major symptoms in addition to joint inflammation are fever, fatigue, headache and rash. The joint symptoms may persist for weeks, even months [13]. Ockelbo disease is a stinging-fly–transmitted polyarthritis in Scandinavia [21]. However, the mosquitoes are also vectors in this disease. It is reported that the transmission of Ockelbo virus by *Culex pipiens* might be interrupted by a prolonged period of cold weather, while transmission by *Culex torrentium* would continue [22]. According to a recent study by Lundstrom et al. [23], the antibody prevalence rates in the oldest age groups were 20 to 40 times higher than the accumulated life-risk of being diagnosed and reported as an Ockelbo disease patient, suggesting that many cases are asymptomatic and/or unreported. A syndrome with rash, arthralgia and moderate fever reactions is a common manifestation of Ockelbo disease [23]. Indirect immunofluorescence and mixed hemadsorption technique to detect viral antibody are the laboratory diagnosis techniques [24]. Considering Karelian fever, *Aedes* species mosquitoes are the vector. This disease was first reported in 1983 [25]. *Aedes communis* is the most common vector [26]. Symptoms including severe arboviral arthritis can be seen.

O'nyong-nyong Virus Infection

O'nyong-nyong virus infection is an arboviral infection. *Aedes* and *Anopheles* mosquitoes are the main vectors. Mansonia can also be the vector. It has been seen in Africa for many decades [27-28]. O'nyong-nyong (ONN) fever, an acute, nonfatal illness characterized by polyarthralgia, is caused by infection with a mosquito-borne central African alphavirus [29-30]. In most cases, articular manifestations involve arthralgia or transient arthritis and are usually minor [29]. An acute febrile illness with polyarthralgia is the most common manifestation in symptomatic cases [30]. According to a recent epidemic in Uganda, among confirmed cases, the knees and ankles were the joints most commonly affected. The median duration of arthralgia was six days and immobilization was four days [31]. In the majority, generalized skin rash was reported, and nearly half had lymphadenopathy, mainly of the cervical region [31]. Although these joint symptoms may be severe and persist for weeks or months in a subacute mode with slight inflammatory episodes that can be relieved using analgesics, they never cause permanent damage [29].

Mayaro Virus Infection

This arboviral arthritis can be seen in South America. *Haemagogus janthinomys* is the principal vector of Mayaro virus and marmosets are the main amplifying hosts [32]. Barroso et al. found that creatine kinase 2 activity in host cells is required in the Mayaro virus infection cycle [33]. According to the findings gathered from a recent epidemic in Brazil, arthralgia was present in virtually all confirmed cases and persisted in some for at least two months, although with decreasing severity [34]. Rash was present in two-thirds of the cases, and was either maculopapular or micropapular and the incidence of rash was higher in children than in adults [34]. Contrary to arthralgia, rash usually appeared on the fifth day and faded within three to four days [34]. In addition, fever, chills, headache, myalgia, lymphadenopathy and other minor clinical manifestations were also recorded [34]. Rebello et al. noted that interferon could inhibit Mayaro virus morphogenesis and the release of virions from cells [35]. The sensitivity of Mayaro virus to interferon-treated cell cultured is confirmed [35-36]. However, interferon is still not the standard therapeutic protocol for Mayaro virus infection. Recently, new trials on prostaglandin [37] and brefeldin [38] on inhibition of Mayaro virus were reported and could be the base for further drug development for treatment of this infection.

References

[1] Russell RC. Mosquito-borne arboviruses in Australia: the current scene and implications of climate change for human health. *Int. J. Parasitol.* 28, 955-69 (1998)

[2] Harley D, Ritchie S, Bain C, Sleigh AC. Risks for Ross River virus disease in tropical Australia. *Int. J. Epidemiol.* (2005)

[3] Kelly-Hope LA, Purdie DM, Kay BH. El Nino Southern Oscillation and Ross River virus outbreaks in Australia. *Vector. Borne. Zoonotic. Dis.* 4, 210-3 (2004)

[4] Kelly-Hope LA, Purdie DM, Kay BH. Differences in climatic factors between Ross River virus disease outbreak and nonoutbreak years. *J. Med. Entomol.* 41, 1116-22 (2004)

[5] Condon RJ, Rouse IL. Acute symptoms and sequelae of Ross River virus infection in South-Western Australia: A follow-up study. *Clin. Diagn. Virol.* 3, 273-84 (1995)

[6] Suhrbier A, La Linn M. Clinical and pathologic aspects of arthritis due to Ross River virus and other alphaviruses. *Curr. Opin. Rheumatol.* 16, 374-9 (2004)

[7] Oliveira NM, Broom AK, Lindsay MD, Mackenzie JS, Kay BH, Hall RA. Specific enzyme immunoassays for the rapid detection of Ross River virus in cell cultures inoculated with infected mosquitoes homogenates. *Clin. Diagn. Virol.* 4,195-205 (1995)

[8] Sellner LN, Coelen RJ, Mackenzie JS. Detection of Ross River virus in clinical samples using a nested reverse transcription-polymerase chain reaction. *Clin. Diagn. Virol.* 4, 257-67 (1995)

[9] Boyd AM, Kay BH. Vector competence of Aedes aegypti, Culex sitiens, Culex annulirostris, and Culex quinquefasciatus (Diptera: Culicidae) for Barmah Forest virus. *J. Med. Entomol.* 37, 660-3 (2000)

[10] Doggett SL, Russell RC, Clancy J, Haniotis J, Cloonan MJ. Barmah Forest virus epidemic on the south coast of New South Wales, Australia, 1994-1995: viruses, vectors, human cases, and environmental factors. *J. Med. Entomol.* 36,:861-8 (1999)

[11] Dore A, Auld J. Barmah Forest viral exanthems. *Australas. J. Dermatol.* 45,125-9 (2004)

[12] Flexman JP, Smith DW, Mackenzie JS, Fraser JR, Bass SP, Hueston L, Lindsay MD, Cunningham AL. A comparison of the diseases caused by Ross River virus and Barmah Forest virus. *Med. J. Aust.* 169, 159-63 (1998)

[13] Laine M, Luukkainen R, Toivanen A. Sindbis viruses and other alphaviruses as cause of human arthritic disease. *J. Intern. Med.* 256, 457-71 (2004)

[14] Kurkela S, Manni T, Myllynen J, Vaheri A, Vapalahti O. Clinical and laboratory manifestations of Sindbis virus infection: prospective study, Finland, 2002-2003. J Infect Dis. 2005 Jun 1;191(11):1820-9.

[15] Kurkela S, Manni T, Vaheri A, Vapalahti O. Causative agent of Pogosta disease isolated from blood and skin lesions. *Emerg. Infect. Dis.* 10, 889-94 (2004)

[16] Laine M, Vainionpaa R, Uksila J, Oksi J, Nissila M, Kaarela K, Luukkainen R, Toivanen A. Prevalence of Sindbis-related (Pogosta) virus infections in patients with arthritis. *Clin. Exp. Rheumatol.* 21, 213-6 (2003)

[17] Turunen M, Kuusisto P, Uggeldahl PE, Toivanen A. Pogosta disease: clinical observations during an outbreak in the province of North Karelia, Finland. *Br. J. Rheumatol.* 37, 1177-80 (1998)

[18] Brummer-Korvenkontio M, Vapalahti O, Kuusisto P, Saikku P, Manni T, Koskela P, Nygren T, Brummer-Korvenkontio H, Vaheri A. Epidemiology of Sindbis virus infections in Finland 1981-96: possible factors explaining a peculiar disease pattern. *Epidemiol. Infect.* 129, 335-45 (2002)

[19] Huang HV. Sindbis virus vectors for expression in animal cells. *Curr. Opin. Biotechnol.* 7, 531-5 (1996)

[20] Hay JG. Sindbis virus--an effective targeted cancer therapeutic. *Trends. Biotechnol.* 22, 501-3 (2004)

[21] Pfeffer M, Dobler G, Hassler D, Lundstrom JO. Ockelbo disease: stinging fly transmitted polyarthritis in Scandinavia. *Dtsch. Med. Wochenschr.* 132, 656-8 (2007)

[22] Lundstrom JO, Vene S, Espmark A, Engvall M, Niklasson B. Effect of environmental temperature on the vector competence of Culex pipiens and Cx. torrentium for Ockelbo virus. *Am. J. Trop. Med. Hyg.* 43, 534-42 (1990)

[23] Lundstrom JO, Vene S, Espmark A, Engvall M, Niklasson B. Geographical and temporal distribution of Ockelbo disease in Sweden. *Epidemiol. Infect.* 106, 567-74 (1991)

[24] Espmark A, Niklasson B. Ockelbo disease in Sweden: epidemiological, clinical, and virological data from the 1982 outbreak. *Am. J. Trop. Med. Hyg.* 33, 1203-11 (1984)

[25] Vershinskii BV, L'vov DK, Skvortsova TM, Kondrashina NG, Lesnikov AL. Karelian fever--a new nosological form of arbovirus etiology (togaviridae, alphavirus, Sindbis complex). *Tr. Inst. Im. Pastera.* 60:31-5 (1983)
[26] Lvov DK, Skvortsova TM, Berezina LK, Gromashevsky VL, Yakovlev BI, Gushchin BV, Aristova VA, Sidorova GA, Gushchina EL, Klimenko SM, et al. Isolation of Karelian fever agent from Aedes communis mosquitoes. *Lancet.* 2, 399-400 (1984)
[27] Williams MC, Woodall JP, Gillett JD. O'nyong-nyong fever: an epidemic virus disease in East Africa. VII. Virus isolation from man and serological studies up to July 1961. *Trans. R. Soc. Trop. Med. Hyg.* 59, 186-97 (1965)
[28] Williams MC, Woodall JP, Corbet PS, Gillett JD. O'nyong-nyong fever: an epidemic virus disease in East Africa. 8. virus isolation from anopheles mosquitoes. *Trans. R. Soc. Trop. Med. Hyg.* 59, 300-6 (1965)
[29] Jeandel P, Josse R, Durand JP. Exotic viral arthritis: role of alphavirus. *Med. Trop.* (Mars). 64, 81-8 (2004)
[30] Sanders EJ, Rwaguma EB, Kawamata J, Kiwanuka N, Lutwama JJ, Ssengooba FP, Lamunu M, Najjemba R, Were WA, Bagambisa G, Campbell GL. O'nyong-nyong fever in south-central Uganda, 1996-1997: description of the epidemic and results of a household-based seroprevalence survey. *J. Infect. Dis.* 180, 1436-43 (1999)
[31] Kiwanuka N, Sanders EJ, Rwaguma EB, Kawamata J, Ssengooba FP, Najjemba R, Were WA, Lamunu M, Bagambisa G, Burkot TR, Dunster L, Lutwama JJ, Martin DA, Cropp CB, Karabatsos N, Lanciotti RS, Tsai TF, Campbell GL. O'nyong-nyong fever in south-central Uganda, 1996-1997: clinical features and validation of a clinical case definition for surveillance purposes. *Clin. Infect. Dis.* 29, 1243-50 (1999)
[32] Hoch AL, Peterson NE, LeDuc JW, Pinheiro FP. An outbreak of Mayaro virus disease in Belterra, Brazil. III. Entomological and ecological studies. *Am. J. Trop. Med. Hyg.* 30, 689-98 (1981)
[33] Barroso MM, Lima CS, Silva-Neto MA, Da Poian AT. Mayaro virus infection cycle relies on casein kinase 2 activity. *Biochem. Biophys. Res. Commun.* 296, 1334-9 (2002)
[34] Pinheiro FP, Freitas RB, Travassos da Rosa JF, Gabbay YB, Mello WA, LeDuc JW. An outbreak of Mayaro virus disease in Belterra, Brazil. I. Clinical and virological findings. *Am. J. Trop. Med. Hyg.* 30, 674-81 (1981)
[35] Rebello MC, Fonseca ME, Marinho JO, Rebello MA. Interferon action on Mayaro virus replication. *Acta. Virol.* 37, 223-31 (1993)
[36] Rebello MC, Fonseca ME, Marinho JO, Rebello MA. Studies on the replication of Mayaro virus grown in interferon treated cells. *Mem. Inst. Oswaldo. Cruz.* 89, 619-23 (1994)
[37] Ishimaru D, Marcicano FG, Rebello MA. Inhibition of Mayaro virus replication by prostaglandin A1 and B2 in Vero cells. *Braz. J. Med. Biol. Res.* 31, 1119-23 (1998)
[38] Da Costa LJ, Rebello MA. Effect of brefeldin A on Mayaro virus replication in Aedes albopictus and Vero cells. *Acta. Virol.* 43, 357-60 (1999)

Chapter XIV

Application of Arbovirus in Gene Medicine

Arbovirus and Gene Transfer

Arbovirus can be used for gene transfer and can act as a vector for gene transfer. For example, vectors derived from South African Arbovirus No. 86 (S.A.AR86) have been proposed [1]. Based on sequence comparisons, S.A.AR86 is in a subgroup of the Sindbis-group viruses that also includes Girdwood S.A. and Ockelbo viruses [1]. The persistence of S.A.AR86 vectors in the cells of the bone, bone marrow, and bone-associated connective tissue can be advantageous for producing an immune response or for methods of therapeutic gene delivery to the cells of the bone and bone marrow, as well as bone-associated connective tissue and neurons [1].

In addition to Sindbis virus, Venezuelan equine encephalitis virus is another simple, enveloped plus-strand RNA virus belonging to the *Alphavirus* genus of the *Togaviridae* family [2]. It is successfully developed into expression vectors that infect a wide host cell range and cause rapid and high-level transgene expression [2]. Due to easy and rapid generation, classification into biosafety levels 1 and 2, and preferential transduction of neurons in cell and tissue cultures makes both Sindbis virus and Venezuelan equine encephalitis virus an increasingly used gene transfer system [2]. Compared to other viral vectors, their advantages include easy and rapid generation of recombinant viral particles, rapid onset, and high-level transgene expression [3]. When applied to neuronal tissue, these vectors possess the additional advantage of efficiently and preferentially transducing neurons rather than non-neuronal cells [3]. However, their main limitation arises from infection-associated cytotoxicity, attributed largely to a progressive shutdown of host cell protein synthesis [4]. Recently, Kim et al. constructed an optimized helper vector, termed DH-BB(tRNA/TE12), for production of SINrep(nsP2S(726)) viral particles with low levels of helper RNA co-packaging and high neurospecificity of infection [4]. Kim noted that SINrep(nsP2S726) is a useful tool for rapid heterologous expression with attenuated cytotoxicity in neurons [4]. In vivo injection of Sindbis virus is confirmed for its effectiveness in rat models [5]. Now it is accepted that virus mediated gene transfer into neurons is a powerful tool for the analysis of neuronal structure and function [5]. Gwag et al. noted that recombinant defective Sindbis viruses can be used as an efficient and selective vector for gene transfer into neurons and applied to investigate the biological role of target genes delivered into neurons in vitro and in vivo [6].

In addition to neurons, Sindbis virus vector is also tested for gene transfer to cardiomyocytes. Basically, somatic gene therapy as a potential strategy for the treatment of myocardial diseases relies on an efficient gene transfer into cardiac muscle cells [7]. The difficulty of delivering genes into adult cardiomyocytes exists not only in vivo but also in primary culture systems [7]. Datwyler et al. reported that Sindbis virus vectors were useful for gene delivery into adult cardiomyocytes and believed that improved versions of this viral system may be useful for cardiovascular gene therapy [7]. Datwyler et al. also demonstrated that the Sindbis virus expression system made possible the straightforward analysis of the localization of sarcomeric proteins in cultured cardiomyocytes and may offer new possibilities for the characterization of mutant proteins involved in hypertrophic cardiomyopathies [8]. According to their study, two recombinant Sindbis viruses were generated, one encoding the myosin-light chain MLC3f-eGFP fusion protein (SINrep5/MLC3f-eGFP), and the other encoding the alpha-actinin-DsRed fusion protein (SINrep5/alpha-actinin-DsRed) [8]. After infection of long-term cultured neonatal and adult rat cardiomyocytes with SINrep5/MLC3f-eGFP, the exogenous MLC3f-eGFP fusion protein localized to the sarcomeres and freshly isolated rod-shaped ventricular cardiomyocytes infected with SINrep5/alpha-actinin-DsRed exhibited a correct incorporation of the newly synthesized alpha-actinin-DsRed fusion protein at the Z-band of the sarcomere [8].

In addition to Sindbis virus vector, Semliki Forest virus vectors are applied for large-scale production of recombinant membrane proteins for drug screening purposes and structural biology studies [9]. Semliki Forest virus is a mosquito borne virus found in Europe. It is now widely used in gene transfer [10-12]. Rapidly generated high-titer Semliki Forest virus vectors can infect numerous mammalian cell lines and primary cell cultures, and result in high levels of transgene expression [13]. Semliki Forest virus-based expression of transmembrane receptors has been characterized by specific ligand-binding activity and functional responses [13]. Adaptation of the Semliki Forest virus technology for mammalian suspension cultures has allowed the production of proteins as previously mentioned [13]. The Semliki Forest virus vectors are confirmed for gene transfer into neurons. Recently, Lundstrom et al. modified the nonstructural protein-2 (nsP2) gene in the Semliki Forest virus vector, pSFV1 [14]. Packaging of Semliki Forest virus replicons with two point mutations in nsP2 resulted in high-titer recombinant Semliki Forest virus (PD) particles [14]. However, Lingor et al. said that the use of novel Semliki Forest virus (PD) vectors was currently limited by persistent neurotoxicity of the vector system [15]. They noted that although Semliki Forest virus (PD) vectors might be useful for protein localization studies in dopaminergic neurons, functional applications will require the development of even less cytopathic vector systems [15]. At present, the main use of Semliki Forest virus in gene transfer is for production of retrovirus-like particles [16].

Arbovirus and Gene Therapy

In addition to gene transfer, many arboviruses can be applied for novel gene therapy. Semliki Forest virus is the one that is widely used for gene therapy. The CNS gene therapy by Semliki Forest virus is widely studied. Tuittila et al. noted that induction of proinflammatory cytokine mRNA in the CNS by SFV infection seemed to correlate with the rate of viral replication and was not significantly influenced by the virus envelope or nonstructural protein primary structure Semliki Forest virus [17]. They said that the results had relevance for development of CNS gene therapy vectors, as SFV4 and A774 display differences in CNS infection characteristics [17]. However, Graham et al. reported that the current SFV1 vector system was limited in its potential for CNS gene therapy by neurotoxicity [18]. In addition to CNS gene therapy, the use of Semliki Forest virus in cancer gene therapy is widely discussed. Lundstrom said that recombinant particles, naked RNA and plasmid DNA containing Semliki Forest virus replicons, demonstrate a strong immune response against recombinantly expressed proteins, which has shown protection against tumor challenges [16]. Intratumoural injection of Semliki Forest virus particles has resulted in tumor regression [16]. Colmenero et al. reported that immunotherapy with recombinant Semliki Forest virus-replicons expressing the P815A tumor antigen or interleukin-12 (IL-12) could induce tumor regression [19]. Murphy et al. reported an inhibition of human lung carcinoma cell growth by apoptosis induction using Semliki Forest virus recombinant particles [20]. In their study [20], direct injection of rSFV into H358a tumours subcutaneously implanted as xenografts in nu/nu mice inhibited tumor growth, and in some cases caused complete regression [20]. It is concluded that tumor growth suppression induced by rSFV was due to apoptosis induction and that the vector has an inherent cell-death–promoting and antitumor activity [20]. Asselin-Paturel et al. reported that transfer of the murine interleukin-12 gene in vivo by a Semliki Forest virus vector could induce B16 tumor regression through inhibition of tumor blood vessel formation monitored by Doppler ultrasonography [21]. In 2007, Lyons et al. reported a similar observation in their study that active immunization with rSFV particles coding for VEGFR-2 could break immunological tolerance and could potentially be used as part of a novel treatment for cancer [22]. They reported that co-immunization of mice with rSFV particles encoding vascular endothelial growth factor receptor-2 (VEGFR-2) and IL-12 completely abrogated both the antibody response and the antitumor effect [22]. It has been proposed that the inhibition of angiogenesis by a Semliki Forest virus vector expressing VEGFR-2 reduces tumour growth and metastasis in mice [22]. This result is similar to a report by Chikkanna-Gowda et al. in 2005 [23]. Indeed, the induction of a therapeutic antitumor immunological response by intratumoral injection of genetically engineered Semliki Forest virus to produce IL-12 has been reported by Yamanaka et al. since 2000 [24].

Sindbis virus is also proposed for its effectiveness in cancer gene therapy [25]. Hay noted that a recent report demonstrates that the Sindbis virus had remarkable properties in three challenging areas of gene therapy specificity, efficacy and delivery, suggesting that Sindbis had the potential to become an important gene therapy vector for cancer therapy [25]. Cancer immunotherapy by Sindbis virus is the new hope in treatment of cancer. Cheng et al. recently used the replication-defective vaccine vector Sindbis virus replicon particles from a new packaging cell line (PCL) to develop Sindbis virus replicon particles encoding calreticulin

(CRT) linked to a model tumor antigen, HPV16 E7 protein [26]. Cheng et al. created a recombinant Sindbis virus-based replicon particle encoding VP22 linked to a model tumor antigen, human papillomavirus type 16 (HPV-16) E7, using a stable SIN PCL [27]. According to this study, Sindbis virus replicon particles encoding calreticulin linked to a tumor antigen generated long-term tumor-specific immunity [26]. Cheng et al. concluded that the CRT strategy used in the context of SIN replicon particles facilitated the generation of a highly effective vaccine for cancer prophylaxis and immunotherapy [26]. Cheng et al. also indicated that the VP22—a herpes simplex virus type 1 (HSV-1) —tegument protein strategy used in the context of Sindbis virus replicon particles may facilitate the generation of a highly effective vaccine for widespread immunization [27]. Zhnag et al. reasoned that Sindbis-virus–based vectors might be ideal for gibbon ape leukemia virus envelope glycoprotein (GALV.fus) gene transfer because high-titer stocks can easily be generated in hamster cells, and Sindbis virus efficiently infects human tumor cells through the high-affinity 67 kDa laminin receptor [28]. They reported that Sindbis vectors expressing GALV.fus could be packaged into infectious viral particles at high levels, exhibiting potent bystander cytopathic potential and were active against U87 glioma xenografts [28]. They concluded that Sindbis-virus-based replicons appeared to be efficient vector systems for delivery and expression of fusogenic membrane glycoproteins [28]. In 1998, Swai and Meruelo explored the possibility of designing a Sindbis virus vector that could target human choriocarcinoma cells via ligand-receptor interaction [29]. In this study, the hCG-envelope chimeric virus vector had minimal infectivities against BHK cells and human cancer cells that did not contain LH/CG receptors on their surface [29]. Swai and Meruelo proposed that the chimeric Sindbis virus vector may provide a novel approach for gene therapy of gestational trophoblast disease and placental dysfunction [29]. Bergman attempted to create a virus that was targeted specifically to breast cancer cells [30]. In their attempt, nonreplicating and replicating pseudotype vesicular stomatitis virus (VSV) was created whose only surface glycoprotein (gp) was a Sindbis gp, called Sindbis-ZZ, modified to severely reduce its native binding function and to contain the Fc-binding domain of *Staphylococcus aureus* protein A [30]. Bergman et al. reported that vesicular stomatitis virus expressing a chimeric Sindbis glycoprotein containing an Fc antibody binding domain could target Her2/neu overexpressing breast cancer cells [30]. This work demonstrates the ability to easily create, directly from plasmid components, an oncolytic replicating VSV with a restricted host cell range [30]. Morizono et al. reported successful targeting in a living animal through intravenous injection of a lentiviral vector pseudotyped with a modified chimeric Sindbis virus envelope (termed m168) [31]. They found that m168 pseudotypes had high titer and high targeting specificity and, unlike other retroviral pseudotypes, had low nonspecific infectivity in the liver and spleen [31]. According to this study, human P-glycoprotein was ectopically expressed on the surface of melanoma cells and targeted by the m168 pseudotyped lentiviral vector conjugated with an antibody specific for P-glycoprotein. The m168 pseudotypes successfully targeted metastatic melanoma cells growing in the lung after systemic administration by tail vein injection [31].

Arbovirus and Vaccine Manipulation

As previously mentioned, many arboviruses can be used as vectors for gene delivery. An important application of this useful delivery property is the design of new vaccines. In 2000, Polo et al. developed plasmid DNA and recombinant vector particle delivery systems derived from the Sindbis virus [32]. Each system uses RNA polymerase II-based expression of viral genome components, and both vector formats are highly efficacious towards inducing robust antigen-specific immune responses in vaccinated animals [32]. In 2004, Leitner et al. showed for the first time that the induction of apoptotic cell death of transfected cells in vivo was required for the increased effectiveness of replicase-based vaccines [33]. Their findings also provided an explanation for the paradoxical observation that replicase-based DNA vaccines are much more immunogenic than conventional constructs, despite reduced antigen production [33]. Leitner et al. noted that arboviral replicons could increase the efficacy and immunogenicity of naked nucleic acid vaccines [33]. Perri et al. said that arboviral replicon particle chimera derived from Venezuelan equine encephalitis and Sindbis viruses was a potent gene-based vaccine delivery vector [34]. According to their study, comparing the replicons with respect to heterologous gene expression levels and sensitivity to alpha/beta interferon in cultured cells indicated that each might contribute to potency differences [34]. This work shows that combining desirable elements from Venezuelan equine encephalitis and Sindbis viruses into a replicon particle chimera may be a valuable approach toward the goal of developing vaccine vectors with optimal in vivo potency, ease of production, and safety [34]. There are many reports on the use of arboviral-related vaccine technology in vaccine development for presently untreatable diseases such as human immunodeficiency virus (HIV) infection and cancer. For a cancer vaccine, examples are also given under the gene therapy heading. In 2005, Otten et al. evaluated the technologies for increasing the potency of HIV DNA vaccines in rhesus macaques [35]. They found that the DNA-based Sindbis virus RNA replicons replicon (pSINCP) vaccines encoding HIV Gag and Env were approximately equal in potency to human cytomegalovirus (CMV) promoter-driven conventional DNA vaccines (pCMV) [35]. They also found that the PLG microparticle DNA delivery system was particularly effective at enhancing antibody responses induced by both pCMV and pSINCP vaccines and had less effect on T cells [35]. Vajdi et al. reported that after vaginal or rectal immunization with Sindbis-Gag and vaginal challenge with vaccinia virus expressing HIV-1 Gag (VV-Gag), despite lower local CD8+ T cell-mediated responses in the vaginal mucosa and iliac lymph nodes, the mice were protected against VV-Gag replication in the ovaries; therefore, local immunization with Sindbis-Gag induced both local mucosal cell-mediated responses and protection [36].

References

[1] Vectors derived from South African Arbovirus No. 86. Available online at http://www.patentstorm.us/patents/6982087-description.html

[2] Ehrengruber MU. Alphaviral gene transfer in neurobiology. *Brain. Res. Bull.* 59, 13-22 (2002)

[3] Ehrengruber MU. Alphaviral vectors for gene transfer into neurons. *Mol. Neurobiol.* 26, 183-201 (2002)

[4] Kim J, Dittgen T, Nimmerjahn A, Waters J, Pawlak V, Helmchen F, Schlesinger S, Seeburg PH, Osten P. Sindbis vector SINrep(nsP2S726): a tool for rapid heterologous expression with attenuated cytotoxicity in neurons. *J. Neurosci. Methods.* 133, 81-90 (2004)

[5] D'Apuzzo M, Mandolesi G, Reis G, Schuman EM. Abundant GFP expression and LTP in hippocampal acute slices by in vivo injection of sindbis virus. *J. Neurophysiol.* 86, 1037-42 (2001)

[6] Gwag BJ, Kim EY, Ryu BR, Won SJ, Ko HW, Oh YJ, Cho YG, Ha SJ, Sung YC. A neuron-specific gene transfer by a recombinant defective Sindbis virus. *Brain. Res. Mol. Brain. Res.* 63, 53-61 (1998)

[7] Datwyler DA, Eppenberger HM, Koller D, Bailey JE, Magyar JP. Efficient gene delivery into adult cardiomyocytes by recombinant Sindbis virus. *J. Mol. Med.* 77, 859-64 (1999)

[8] Datwyler DA, Magyar JP, Busceti V, Hirschy A, Perriard JC, Bailey JE, Eppenberger HM. Recombinant Sindbis virus allows expression and precise targeting of proteins of the contractile apparatus in cultured cardiomyocytes. *Basic. Res. Cardiol.* 96, 630-5 (2001)

[9] Lundstrom K. Biology and application of alphaviruses in gene therapy. *Gene. Ther.* 12 Suppl 1, S92-7 (2005)

[10] Wahlfors J, Morgan RA. Semliki Forest virus vectors for gene transfer. *Methods. Mo.l Med.* 76, 493-502 (2003)

[11] Lundstrom K, Ehrengruber MU. Semliki Forest virus (SFV) vectors in neurobiology and gene therapy. *Methods. Mol. Med.* 76, 503-23 (2003)

[12] Lundstrom K. Semliki Forest virus vectors for large-scale production of recombinant proteins. *Methods. Mol. Med.* 76, 525-43 (2003)

[13] Lundstrom K, Schweitzer C, Rotmann D, Hermann D, Schneider EM, Ehrengruber MU. Semliki Forest virus vectors: efficient vehicles for in vitro and in vivo gene delivery. *FEBS. Lett.* 504, 99-103 (2001)

[14] Lundstrom K, Abenavoli A, Malgaroli A, Ehrengruber MU. Novel Semliki Forest virus vectors with reduced cytotoxicity and temperature sensitivity for long-term enhancement of transgene expression. *Mol. Ther.* 7, 202-9 (2003)

[15] Lingor P, Scholl U, Bahr M, Kugler S. Functional applications of novel Semliki Forest virus vectors are limited by vector toxicity in cultures of primary neurons in vitro and in the substantia nigra in vivo. *Exp. Brain. Res.* 161, 335-42 (2005)

[16] Lundstrom K. Semliki Forest virus vectors for gene therapy. *Expert. Opin. Biol. Ther.* 3, 771-7 (2003)

[17] Tuittila M, Nygardas P, Hinkkanen A. mRNA expression of proinflammatory cytokines in mouse CNS correlates with replication rate of semliki forest virus but not with the strain of viral proteins. *Viral. Immunol.* 17, 287-97 (2004)

[18] Graham A, Walker R, Baird P, Hahn CN, Fazakerley JK. CNS gene therapy applications of the Semliki Forest virus 1 vector are limited by neurotoxicity. *Mol. Ther.* 13, 631-5 (2006)

[19] Colmenero P, Chen M, Castanos-Velez E, Liljestrom P, Jondal M. Immunotherapy with recombinant SFV-replicons expressing the P815A tumor antigen or IL-12 induces tumor regression. *Int. J. Cancer.* 98, 554-60 (2002)

[20] Murphy AM, Morris-Downes MM, Sheahan BJ, Atkins GJ. Inhibition of human lung carcinoma cell growth by apoptosis induction using Semliki Forest virus recombinant particles. *Gene. Ther.* 7, 1477-82 (2000)

[21] Asselin-Paturel C, Lassau N, Guinebretiere JM, Zhang J, Gay F, Bex F, Hallez S, Leclere J, Peronneau P, Mami-Chouaib F, Chouaib S. Transfer of the murine interleukin-12 gene in vivo by a Semliki Forest virus vector induces B16 tumor regression through inhibition of tumor blood vessel formation monitored by Doppler ultrasonography. *Gene. Ther.* 6, 606-15 (1999)

[22] Lyons JA, Sheahan BJ, Galbraith SE, Mehra R, Atkins GJ, Fleeton MN. Inhibition of angiogenesis by a Semliki Forest virus vector expressing VEGFR-2 reduces tumour growth and metastasis in mice. *Gene. Ther.* 14, 503-13 (2007)

[23] Chikkanna-Gowda CP, Sheahan BJ, Fleeton MN, Atkins GJ. Regression of mouse tumours and inhibition of metastases following administration of a Semliki Forest virus vector with enhanced expression of IL-12. *Gene. Ther.* 12, 1253-63 (2005)

[24] Yamanaka R, Zullo SA, Tanaka R, Ramsey J, Blaese M, Xanthopoulos KG. Induction of a therapeutic antitumor immunological response by intratumoral injection of genetically engineered Semliki Forest virus to produce interleukin-12. *Neurosurg. Focus.* 9, e7 (2000)

[25] Hay JG. Sindbis virus--an effective targeted cancer therapeutic. *Trends. Biotechnol.* 22, 501-3 (2004)

[26] Cheng WF, Lee CN, Su YN, Chai CY, Chang MC, Polo JM, Hung CF, Wu TC, Hsieh CY, Chen CA. Sindbis virus replicon particles encoding calreticulin linked to a tumor antigen generate long-term tumor-specific immunity. *Cancer. Gene. Ther.* 13, 873-85 (2006)

[27] Cheng WF, Hung CF, Hsu KF, Chai CY, He L, Polo JM, Slater LA, Ling M, Wu TC. Cancer immunotherapy using Sindbis virus replicon particles encoding a VP22-antigen fusion. *Hum.Gene. Ther.* 13, 553-68 (2002)

[28] Zhang J, Frolov I, Russell SJ. Gene therapy for malignant glioma using Sindbis vectors expressing a fusogenic membrane glycoprotein. *J. Gene. Med.* 6, 1082-91 (2004)

[29] Sawai K, Meruelo D. Cell-specific transfection of choriocarcinoma cells by using Sindbis virus hCG expressing chimeric vector. *Biochem. Biophys. Res. Commun.* 248, 315-23 (1998)

[30] Bergman I, Whitaker-Dowling P, Gao Y, Griffin JA, Watkins SC. Vesicular stomatitis virus expressing a chimeric Sindbis glycoprotein containing an Fc antibody binding domain targets to Her2/neu overexpressing breast cancer cells. *Virology.* 316, 337-47 (2003)

[31] Morizono K, Xie Y, Ringpis GE, Johnson M, Nassanian H, Lee B, Wu L, Chen IS. Lentiviral vector retargeting to P-glycoprotein on metastatic melanoma through intravenous injection. *Nat. Med.* 11, 346-52 (2005)

[32] Polo JM, Gardner JP, Ji Y, Belli BA, Driver DA, Sherrill S, Perri S, Liu MA, Dubensky TW Jr. Alphavirus DNA and particle replicons for vaccines and gene therapy. *Dev. Biol. (Basel).* 104, 181-5 (2000)

[33] Leitner WW, Hwang LN, Bergmann-Leitner ES, Finkelstein SE, Frank S, Restifo NP. Apoptosis is essential for the increased efficacy of alphaviral replicase-based DNA vaccines. *Vaccine.* 22, 1537-44 (2004)

[34] Perri S, Greer CE, Thudium K, Doe B, Legg H, Liu H, Romero RE, Tang Z, Bin Q, Dubensky TW Jr, Vajdy M, Otten GR, Polo JM. An alphavirus replicon particle chimera derived from venezuelan equine encephalitis and sindbis viruses is a potent gene-based vaccine delivery vector. *J. Virol.* 77, 10394-403 (2003)

[35] Otten GR, Schaefer M, Doe B, Liu H, Srivastava I, Megede J, Kazzaz J, Lian Y, Singh M, Ugozzoli M, Montefiori D, Lewis M, Driver DA, Dubensky T, Polo JM, Donnelly J, O'Hagan DT, Barnett S, Ulmer JB. Enhanced potency of plasmid DNA microparticle human immunodeficiency virus vaccines in rhesus macaques by using a priming-boosting regimen with recombinant proteins. *J. Virol.* 79, 8189-200 (2005)

[36] Vajdy M, Gardner J, Neidleman J, Cuadra L, Greer C, Perri S, O'Hagan D, Polo JM. Human immunodeficiency virus type 1 Gag-specific vaginal immunity and protection after local immunizations with sindbis virus-based replicon particles. *J. Infect. Dis.* 184, 1613-6 (2001)

Index

A

B

C

D

E

F

G

H

I

J

K

L

M

N

Q

R

S

T

W

X

Y

Z